Reproductive Technologies

READINGS IN BIOETHICS

Edited by Thomas A. Shannon

Readings in Bioethics is a series of anthologies that gather together seminal essays in four areas: reproductive technologies, genetic technologies, death and dying, and health care policy. Each of the readers addresses specific case studies and issues under its respective topic. The goal of this series is twofold: first, to provide a set of readers on thematic topics for introductory or survey courses in bioethics or for courses with a particular theme or time limitation. When used in conjunction with a core text that provides the appropriate level of analytical framework, the readers in this series provide specific analysis of a set of issues that meets the professor's individual needs and interests. Second, each of the readers in this series is designed with the student in mind and aims to present important articles that help students focus more thoroughly and effectively on specific topics that flesh out the ethical issues at the core of bioethics.

Volumes in the Readings in Bioethics Series:

Reproductive Technologies
Genetic Technologies
Death and Dying
Health Care Policy

Reproductive Technologies

A Reader

Edited by
Thomas A. Shannon

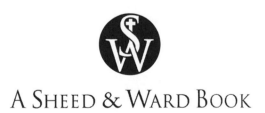

A SHEED & WARD BOOK

ROWMAN & LITTLEFIELD PUBLISHERS, INC.
Lanham • Boulder • New York • Toronto • Oxford

A SHEED & WARD BOOK

ROWMAN & LITTLEFIELD PUBLISHERS, INC.

Published in the United States of America
by Rowman & Littlefield Publishers, Inc.
A wholly owned subsidary of The Rowman & Littlefield Publishing Group, Inc.
4501 Forbes Boulevard, Suite 200, Lanham, Maryland 20706
www.rowmanlittlefield.com

PO Box 317
Oxford
OX2 9RU, UK

British Library Cataloguing in Publication Information Available

Library of Congress Cataloging-in-Publication Data

Reproductive technologies: a reader / [edited by] Thomas A.
Shannon.
    p. cm.—(Readings in bioethics)
"A Sheed & Ward book."
Includes bibliographical references and index. ISBN 0-7425-3150-3 (alk. paper)—
ISBN 0-7425-3151-1 (pbk.: alk. paper)
    1. Reproductive technology—Miscellanea. I. Shannon, Thomas A.
(Thomas Anthony), 1940- II. Series.
RG133.5 .R468 2004
616.6'92—dc22   2003019009

Printed in the United States of America

♾ ™ The paper used in this publication meets the minimum requirements of American
National Standard for Information Sciences—Permanence of Paper for Printed Library
Materials, ANSI/NISO Z39.48-1992.

To Pietro and Isolina Pinto
with much love to you and your family

Contents

Acknowledgments

Gratefully acknowledged are the publishers and authors of the works listed below for their permission to reprint their publications.

David Adamson. "Regulation of Assisted Reproductive Technologies in the United States." *Fertility and Sterility* 78 (November 2002): 932–42. Reprinted by permission of the American Society for Reproductive Medicine.

James P. Toner. "Progress We Can Be Proud Of: U.S. Trends in Assisted Reproduction Over the First 20 Years." *Fertility and Sterility* 78 (November 2002): 943–50. Reprinted by permission of the American Society for Reproductive Medicine.

Thomas A. Shannon. "Reproductive Technologies: Ethical and Religious Issues." In *God Forbid: Religion and Sex in American Public Life*. Ed. Kathleen Sands. Oxford University Press, 2000, 203–18. Reprinted by Permission of Oxford University Press, Inc.

Bonnie Steinbock. "Sex Selection: Not Obviously Wrong." *Hastings Center Report* 32 (January–February 2002): 23–28. Reprinted by permission of the *Hastings Center Report*.

Ethics Committee of the American Society for Reproductive Medicine. "Human Immunodeficiency Virus and Infertility Treatment." *Fertility and Sterility* 77 (February 2002): 218–22. Reprinted by permission of the American Society for Reproductive Medicine

Laura A. Schieve, Susan F. Meikle, Cynthia Ferre, Herbert B. Peterson, Gary Jeng, and Lynne S. Wilcox. "Low and Very Low Birth Weight in Infants Conceived with Use of Assisted Reproductive Technology." *The New England Journal of Medicine* 346 (March 7, 2002): 731–37. Copyright © 2002 by Massachusetts Medical Society. All rights reserved. Reprinted by permission.

Richard J. Paulson, Robert Boostanfar, Peyman Saadat, Eliran Mor, David E. Tourgeman, Cristin C. Slater, Mary M. Francis, and John K. Jain. "Pregnancy in the Sixth Decade of Life: Obstetric Outcomes in Women of Advanced Reproductive Age." *The Journal of the American Medical Association* 288 (November 13, 2002): 2320–23. Reprinted by permission of the American Medical Society.

G. Pennings. "Reproductive Tourism as Moral Pluralism in Motion." *Journal of Medical Ethics* 28 (2002): 337–41. Reprinted by Permission of the British Medical Journal Publishing (BMJ) Group.

Thomas H. Murray. "What Are Families For? Getting to an Ethics of Reproductive Technology." *Hastings Center Report* 32 (May–June 2002): 41–45. Reprinted by permission of the *Hastings Center Report*.

Lori B. Andrews. "Mom, Dad, Clone: Implications for Reproductive Privacy." *Cambridge Quarterly of Healthcare Ethics* 7 (1998): 176–186. Reprinted by Permission of Cambridge University Press.

J. M. Phillips. "Cloned Child." *America* (November 25, 2000): 13. Reprinted by Permission of America Press.

Editor's Introduction

Since its introduction over a decade ago, the field of bioethics has grown exponentially. Not only has it become established as an academic discipline with journals and professional societies, it is covered regularly in the media and affects people everyday around the globe.

One important development in the field has been the informal division into clinical and institutional bioethics. Institutional bioethics has to do with the ethical dilemmas associated with the various institutions, the majority of which are providers of health care services. Delivery of health care, allocations of health care payments, mergers, closing or restricting services of certain departments or even of hospitals or clinics themselves are systemic questions involving a broad range of ethical agenda. On the clinical side, the bevy of usual suspects of ethical dilemmas is increasing in complexity as technology moves forward, new interventions are proposed, and fantasies become realities. Few, for example, thought that human cloning would become a serious clinical, public policy, and institutional debate in 2002.

One of the major consequences of this quantitative and qualitative debate is that providing resources for introductory or even specialized courses is becoming much more difficult. This is particularly difficult in the case of editing an anthology to compliment a text that provides an analysis of the core ethical issues. There is simply too much material to put into a single anthology that is reasonable in price and convenient in size.

This series is an attempt to resolve the problem of a cumbersome and expensive anthology by providing a set of four manageable and accessible readers on specific topics. Thus each reader in the series will be on a specific topic—reproductive technologies, genetic technologies, death and dying, and health care policy—and will be about two hundred pages in length. This is to provide professors with flexibility in designing their courses. Ideally, professors will use a core text to analyze the primary ethical issues in bioethics and will use the readers in this series to examine specific problems and cases, thus providing flexibility in designing syllabi as well as providing variety in presenting the course.

The goal of this series is twofold: first, to provide a set of readers on thematic topics for introductory or survey courses in bioethics or for courses with a particular theme or time limitation. In addition to a core text that provides the appropriate level of analytical framework, the readers in this series provide specific analysis of a set of issues that meets the professor's needs and interests. Second, each of the readers in this series is designed with the student in mind and aims to present seminal articles and case studies that help students focus more thoroughly and effectively on specific topics that flesh out the ethical issues at the core of bioethics.

1

Regulation of Assisted Reproductive Technologies in the United States

David Adamson

There is a widely perceived notion that assisted reproductive technology (ART) is not regulated in the United States. This current perception has developed for a number of reasons.

In the United States, ART has been characterized by the absence of a socialized health-care system, lack of centralized government or financial oversight, and the proliferation of a large number of clinics to meet market demand. Although some of these clinics are based in universities, which are operated under state oversight, and some are in private academic centers, many function as private medical practices.

Second, there is no statutory national body, such as the Reproductive Technology Accreditation Committee (RTAC) in Australia, or the Human Fertilization and Embryology Authority (HFEA) in England, to oversee these programs. (1)

Third, highly publicized incidents of illegal, immoral, irresponsible, and unethical behavior have occurred in the United States in the past few years. Extensive media exposure of physicians using their own semen for patient insemination, theft of patient eggs, proposals for human cloning, the use of stem cells for research, exorbitant sums of money paid to egg donors, and septuplet and octuplet births have received wide media attention. As a result, the perception is that these events represent the norm, rather than anomalous incidents.

Fourth, the rapid pace of scientific advances in ART has led to the use of new techniques such as cryopreservation of eggs, intracytoplasmic sperm injection (ICSI), embryo hatching, sex selection, cytoplasmic transfer, and preimplantation genetic diagnosis in patients before large, well-designed clinical trials have confirmed their safety and efficacy. This has led to criticisms of experimenting on humans in an irresponsible fashion. Furthermore, the political climate surrounding abortion—and, by extension, embryo research,

1

stem cells, and somatic cell nuclear transfer—has, until now, resulted in a vacuum of governmental involvement in ART research.

Finally, the media has perpetuated the current perception of an uncontrolled industry.

Yet, despite its shortcomings, the current regulatory status of ART in the United States is far from laissez faire. Perspective is needed on the issues related to current and potential regulation of ART in the United States. Professional societies and individuals involved with ART have worked with federal and state governments and with professional and other organizations to develop an improved process that should ensure higher quality care, protect the public interest, and create public confidence in ART services.

CURRENT REGULATIONS

Mandatory General Medical Regulations Affecting ART

The federal government has several mandatory regulations affecting medicine in general which also affect the clinical practice of ART. These include the Clinical Laboratory Improvement Amendments of 1988 (CLIA 88) which mandate, among many other requirements, certain standards for andrology laboratories, and also cover those that provide ART services. Strict compliance with standards and on-site inspections are required. The Center for Medicare and Medicaid Services (CMS), formerly Health Care Financing Administration (HCFA), is responsible for approving diagnostic and procedural coding terminology and the resource-based relative value studies (RBRVS) units that determine reimbursement for ART procedures. The Food and Drug Administration (FDA) also has numerous regulations affecting the use of the pharmaceutical products used in ART.

On the state level, a license to practice medicine is required to practice ART and inappropriate activities in ART clinics can and have been investigated by state licensing bodies. Most ART practitioners are certified by the American Board of Obstetrics and Gynecology, and many by the Reproductive Endocrinology Subspecialty Board. However, neither is required to practice ART. Facilities in which ART is practiced, such as hospitals, operating rooms, and procedure rooms, are also strictly licensed and inspected.

At the university level, regulations for clinical research and ethics are in place to protect patients, physicians, and the institutions. Locally, county medical societies, hospitals, and health maintenance organizations (HMOs) usually oversee the practice of medicine and deal with the clinical, financial, and ethical issues brought to them by patients, physicians, or others.

Mandatory Clinical ART-Specific Regulations

The most visible and important ART-specific regulation that has been developed in the United States is the Fertility Clinic Success Rate and Certification Act of 1992 (FCSRCA), sponsored by congressman Ron Wyden. (2) This law requires that "each ART program shall annually report to the Secretary through the Centers for Disease Control and Prevention (CDC) pregnancy success rates achieved by such program through each assisted reproductive technology and the identity of each embryo laboratory used by such program, and whether the laboratory is certified or has applied for such certification." The law calls for the Secretary to consult with appropriate consumer and professional organizations in developing definitions. It also calls for the CDC "to develop a model program for the certification of embryo laboratories . . . to be carried out by the States. In developing the certification program, the Secretary may not establish any regulation, standard or requirement which has the effect of exercising supervision or control over the practice of medicine in ART programs."

The law also calls for the Secretary, through the CDC, to promulgate criteria and procedures for the approval of accreditation organizations to inspect and certify embryo laboratories. The Secretary will also evaluate annually the performance of each accreditation organization. States, or accrediting organizations that issue a certification to an embryo laboratory, also have the right to revoke or suspend the license. The FCSRCA also requires the CDC to publish annually and distribute to the states and to the public the statistics on pregnancy success rates, the programs that have failed to report, and the status of the embryo laboratory's certification. The Secretary may require the payment of fees for the purpose of, and in an amount sufficient to cover the cost of, administering the FRSRCA.

The current status of law is as follows. The law has been enacted and over 95% of ART programs in the country annually report their results to the CDC through the Society for Assisted Reproductive Technology (SART), which has a contract with the CDC to collect these data. Those few programs that elect not to report have their names listed as "non-reporters" in the CDC publication. In 1997, for the first time, the 1995 results were posted on the Internet. Results for 1996 through 1999 are also posted. Also, in 1997 on-site validation inspections were initiated by SART, sometimes with CDC observers, to ensure the accuracy of the data that were reported through SART to the CDC. Thirty clinics of the approximately 370 in the United States had an on-site validation inspection. Programs are selected for a validation inspection based on those with highest and lowest success rates, as well as randomly. (Further comment on the FRSRCA will made later in this paper.)

In addition to the FCSRCA, the National Institutes of Health (NIH) has multiple regulations governing research in reproductive medicine. These laws are also frequently considered in non-NIH funded research. The federal and state governments have also passed laws regarding certain aspects of ART. For example, federal law and several state laws prohibit cloning a human; compensating a gestational carrier is prohibited in Michigan; and cryopreservation is limited on Louisiana. New York State requires licensure of ART laboratories, and California requires a provisional license. (3, 4)

At the university level, many state universities have laws specifically preventing the use of, or research in, certain ART technologies, and ethical oversight by appropriate committees is mandatory for any reproductive research.

Mandatory Nonmedical Regulation of Clinical ART

The Federal Trade Commission (FTC) has regulations regarding truth in advertising and marketing. A number of ART programs in the United States have been investigated by the FTC for making claims about their pregnancy success rates that could not be substantiated by their clinical data. For example, when clinics advertise their success rates, the FTC has required that they must disclose the numerator and the denominator used in their calculations when such advertised rates are not based on initiated cycles and live births. The FTC has the authority to, and has in the past, publicized these transgressions and issued cease and desist orders. They also can impose punitive sanctions such as fines. Working conditions for clinic employees are regulated by the Occupational Safety and Hazard Act (OSHA), which has numerous strict requirements regulating employees in all medical practices, including ART. These regulations can and are enforced by on-site inspections.

State regulations also require a license for business, which includes ART clinics. In local communities, cities and towns require commercial licenses, have building codes for facilities, and have other regulations that affect ART clinics.

Other mandatory nonmedical regulations include insurance company, HMO, and other healthcare organization requirements. In early 1999, Tufts Health Plan in Boston deselected three of nine ART providers based on criteria Tufts Health Plan had set, which included number of physicians, percentage of reproductive endocrinologists, and success rates. Physicians must also follow federal and state laws the same as nonphysicians.

Another most interesting development was the finding by the United States Supreme Court in the case *Bragdon v. Abbott* in June 1998, interdicta, that infertility is a major life activity as defined by the Americans with Disabilities Act (ADA). The short and long-term impact of this finding is as yet unknown, but class action lawsuits based on this finding are in process. The Equal Employment Opportunity Commission (EEOC) also found in a New

York case that failure to provide infertility benefits is discriminatory, although the finding in this case was changed on appeal. National ramifications of these legal and regulatory cases are still being determined in subsequent cases.

Mandatory Laboratory Regulations

As noted above, andrology laboratories are covered under CLIA 88, and when these same laboratories also perform portions of the ART procedure, that portion falls under CLIA 88. The Centers for Medicare and Medicaid Services (CMS) also develops the diagnostic, procedural, and billing codes on a national basis for laboratories. Other national organizations that regulate ART laboratories include the Joint Commission on Accreditation of Healthcare Organizations (JCAHO). This commission has the authority and does inspect some ART laboratories that are located in hospitals.

Some states also have mandatory regulations involving ART laboratories. New York State inspects laboratories, and California ART laboratories currently are provisionally licensed under the California Tissue Bank Licensure Laws. (3, 4)

ART Research Regulations

The history of ART research regulations in the United States has been political and complex. Prior to 1993, federal policy required review and approval of research involving ART by an ethical advisory board (EAB), which had been established in 1975 to oversee research in reproduction. In 1979, the EAB released a report supporting ART research. However, because of the politics surrounding abortion, a chair for the committee could not be agreed upon; thus, the EAB was disbanded in 1980. From 1980 to 1993 federal policy required review and approval of ART research by a board that did not exist. As a result, no research was approved for federal funding.

Recognizing this problem, the federal government established the Human Embryo Research Panel, which in 1993 recommended that some research be acceptable (for example, embryo research up to 14 days) and that other research not be acceptable (for example, cloning). President Clinton immediately tabled this report for further study. Following review, in 1994 a limited approach was taken to the report and a law was passed with a provision not to support "the creation of human embryos for research purposes." Following further study, in 1996 President Clinton signed a "continuing resolution" that banned federal funding for human embryo research. However, in 1999 the NIH initiated requests for proposals (RFP) for reproductive research that could involve embryos; however, embryos could not be created for the research and had to be obtained in the course of clinical care. Such research has to meet very rigorous NIH research guidelines, but represents increasing recognition of the potential widespread benefits of research in this area. In July 2001, President George W. Bush promulgated regulations under which stem cell research could receive federal funding in the United States.

Mandatory Regulation of Somatic Cell Nuclear Transfer

Somatic cell nuclear transfer (SCNT) has more commonly been termed "cloning" by the media. Since Dolly the cloned sheep came on the international scene in 1997, several controversial bills have been introduced but not passed regarding SCNT. At the height of the controversy over Dolly, Congress came very close to passing restrictive legislation regarding SCNT, but this was forestalled by giving the FDA authority to oversee such programs. In 2001, the House of Representatives approved a ban of both reproductive SCNT ("cloning" of a person) as well as therapeutic SCNT (the production of cells and tissue for the purpose of research and treatment of diseases). The Senate did not pass the bill, so no legislation has yet to result. Senate legislation of this issue has come forward in 2002, but the outcome of the various proposals is currently unknown.

In the interim, the FDA has claimed authority, and has instructed all ART laboratories that FDA permission to perform any type of SCNT is required through the submission of a New Drug Application (NDA). At this time no NDAs have been approved and there is strong indication that the FDA will not give approval for any type of SCNT research. This requirement does not necessarily prevent private entities from performing such research, but federal legislation potentially could.

Mandatory Regulation of Genetics Testing and Treatment

Regulation of genetics is rapidly becoming an integral aspect of regulation of ART. The federal Department of Health and Human Services (DHHS) has oversight authority of genetic tests through the Centers for Disease Control (CDC), Food and Drug Administration (FDA), Centers for Medicare and Medicaid Services (CMS) and Office for Human Research Protection (OHRP). The Clinical Laboratories Improvement Act (CLIA) provides laboratory oversight. The National Institutes of Health (NIH) and other agencies support genetics research activities.

The Secretary's Advisory Committee on Genetic Testing (SACGT) made recommendations in 2000 regarding criteria to assess genetic tests, classification of tests into scrutiny levels, data collection, confidentiality, oversight mechanisms, institution review boards, informed consent, transition of genetic tests to clinical use, orphan diseases, social and ethical concerns, current genetic tests, and regulation enforcement (http://www4.od.nih.gov/oba/sacgt.htm). The Health Care Portability and Accountability Act of 1996 restricts use of genetic test data by health insurers; and Equal Opportunity Commission guidelines prohibit employment discrimination based on genetic tests. Additionally, there is a prohibition on human embryo research (Public Health Service Act (42 U.S.C. 289g(b))).

State health agencies have an oversight role in genetic testing including licensure of personnel and facilities and quality assurance activities under the CLIA program. Some states have additional regulations.

Mandatory Regulation of ART Human Subject Research

The federal government has numerous regulations regarding research involving human subjects that apply regardless of the funding source. Institutional review board (IRB) approval is needed if human research projects are federally funded or will be submitted to the FDA. Written consent of the research participants is always required. The Department of Health and Human Services (DHHS) requires review and approval of research involving human subjects prior to funding by federal agencies. Additionally, university institutional oversight requires that regulations be adhered to and that IRB approval be obtained for research projects.

PROFESSIONAL ACCOMPLISHMENTS THAT HAVE ENHANCED OVERSIGHT OF ART

CAP/ASRM Laboratory Accreditation Program

Numerous initiatives have been taken by professional societies associated with ART in the United States. The American Society for Reproductive Medicine (ASRM) was founded in 1944 and has been actively involved in research, education, and setting standards for practice in reproductive medicine, including ART. Founded in 1987, SART is an affiliate society of the ASRM; it published 1989 clinic-specific success rates on a voluntary basis, and has continued annual publication since then. Both SART and ASRM worked with congressman Wyden to support the FCSRCA, which passed in 1992. (2) With the College of American Pathologists, SART and ASRM also developed the CAP/ASRM Reproductive Laboratory Accreditation Programs (RLAP). (5)

The RLAP includes strict standards collaboratively developed by professionals in the field in 1992, and on-site laboratory inspections by CAP/ASRM/RLAP inspectors. Over 200 SART clinics have now been accredited on a voluntary basis by this national accrediting body. As a result of changes in SART bylaws, in December 1998 accreditation became mandatory for all SART programs; programs must apply for accreditation to CAP/ASRM, JCAHO, or the state of New York. Those IVF clinics that do not become accredited or do not apply for accreditation lose their membership in SART. At this time essentially all SART clinics have completed accreditation or are in the process of completing accreditation.

American Association of Bioanalysts

The American Association of Bioanalysts (AAB) has a proficiency testing service that is approved by CLIA. The AAB also supports CLIA coverage of embryology laboratories, and has a grandfather provision for embryology laboratory directors who do not have doctoral degrees.

Professional Society Guidelines and Practice Standards

The ASRM and SART have collaboratively developed professional society guidelines and practice standards, shown in table 1.1. (6)

The American College of Obstetricians and Gynecologists (ACOG) has also developed technical bulletins and practice opinions on ART procedures (table 1.2). (7)

Professional Society Ethical Guidelines

Recognizing the social context in which ART must be practiced, ASRM, SART, and ACOG have not confined their concerns regarding ART just to the clinical and laboratory practice of medicine. Considerable time, effort, and expertise have been devoted to developing ethical guideline initiatives that have created standards for self-regulation. Because most practitioners follow these guidelines, they have been important in directing the ethical practice of ART (table 1.3). (6, 7)

Recommendations are that preimplantation genetic diagnosis (PGD) to prevent transmission of serious genetic disease, including by sex selection, is ethically acceptable, sex selection during IVF for nonmedical reasons should not be encouraged, initiation of IVF with preimplantation genetic

Table 1.1   ASRM and SART Guidelines and Practice Standards

- Minimum standards for IVF (1984)
- Minimum standards for GIFT (I988)
- Revised minimum standards for IVF, GIFT, and related procedures (1990)
- Guidelines for human embryology and andrology laboratories (1992)
- Guidelines for practice, including gamete donation (1993)
- Statement on intracytoplasmic sperm injection (1994)
- Guidelines for the provision of infertility services (1996)
- Elements to be considered in obtaining informed consent for ART (1997)
- Induction of ovarian follicle development and ovulation with exogenous gonadotropins (1998)
- Guidelines for number of embryos transferred (1998)
- Guidelines for gamete and embryo donation (1998)
- Revised minimum standards for in vitro fertilization, gamete intrafallopian transfer, and related procedures (1998)
- Position statement on nurses performing limited ultrasound in a gynecology/infertility setting (1997)
- Intravenous immunoglobulin (IVIG) and recurrent spontaneous pregnancy loss (1998)
- Guidelines on number of embryos to transfer (1999)
- Antiphospholipid antibodies do not affect IVF success (1999)
- Who is to report ART cycles (1999)
- Optimal evaluation of the infertile female (2000)
- The role of assisted hatching in IVF: a review of the literature (2000)
- Repetitive oocyte donation (2000)
- Does intracytoplasmic sperm injection (ICSI) carry inherent genetic risks? (2000)
- Blastocyst production and transfer in clinical assisted reproduction (2001)
- Salpingectomy for hydrosalpinx prior to IVF (2001)
- Preimplantation genetic diagnosis (2001)

Source: Adamson. Regulation of ART in the U.S. *Fertil Steril* 2002.

diagnosis solely for the purpose of sex selection should be discouraged, and further studies of the consequences of sex selection are needed. The use of somatic cell nuclear transfer for reproduction or producing a "clone" is strongly opposed, whereas the use of SCNT for therapeutic purposes is supported under rigorous research guidelines and oversight.

Table 1.2   ACOG Technical Bulletins and Practice Opinions

- Technical bulletin on infertility (1989)
- Technical bulletin on new reproductive technologies (1990)
- Technical bulletin male infertility (1990)
- Practice opinion on ZIFT (1993)
- Technical bulletin male infertility (1994)
- Practice opinion on use of frozen sperm (1994)

Source: Adamson. Regulation of ART in the U.S. *Fertil Steril* 2002.

Table 1.3   Professional Society Ethical Guidelines

- ASRM and SART: Ethical considerations of the assisted reproductive technologies (1986, 1988, 1990, 1994, 1997)
  - 1994 report with complete statements on over 29 topics
  - 1997 report with statements on:
    - disposition of abandoned embryos
    - oocyte donation to postmenopausal women
    - embryo splitting for intertility treatment
    - the use of fetal oocytes in assisted reproduction
    - posthumous reproduction
    - ASRM and SART: Ethical issues with respect to specific ART practices including IVF, GIFT, ZIFT, gamete donation, surrogacy, cryopreservation of embryos, and research
- ASRM and SART: Guidelines addressing quality assurance and formation of public policy
  - Definition of "experimental" (1993)
  - Definition of "infertility" (1993)
- ACOG committee on ethics, and opinions on IVF (1986), surrogacy (1990) and research on preimplantation embryos (1993)
- The National Advisory Board on Ethics in Reproduction (NABER) [Originally organized through the cooperative efforts of ACOG and ASRM in 1991, then became independently incorporated and funded and had broad representation before disbanding in 1998 because of lack of funding]: Informed consent and the use of gametes and embryos for research (1997)
  - ASRM and SART: Shared-risk or refund programs in assisted reproduction (1998)
  - Guidelines for advertising by ART programs (1998, 1999)
  - Sex selection and preimplantation genetic diagnosis (1999)
  - Financial incentives in recruitment of oocyte donors (2000)
  - Human somatic cell nuclear transfer—cloning (2000)
  - Preconception gender selection for nonmedical reasons (2001)

Source: Adamson. Regulation of ART in the U.S. *Fertil Steril* 2002.

RECENT DEVELOPMENTS IN ART OVERSIGHT IN THE UNITED STATES

ASRM and SART Clinic-Specific Report and Validation Program

The past 4 years have seen a dramatic increase in the pace at which ASRM and SART have been working with other organizations, especially the CDC and RESOLVE, to enhance the collecting, analyzing, and publishing of clinic-specific success rates. (8, 9) Through its registry committee, SART has completely reviewed and refined all of the variables that are collected for the annual report. In addition, a survey of SART members has been taken to help improve the data definition and collection process. Also, the turn-around time for publication of the report has been significantly reduced. Prospective reporting of data is already in place, with full compliance expected in the very near future.

In 1998 SART and ASRM, along with the CDC, developed an on-site validation program. (6) Twenty-five programs were inspected in 1998 and 30 more programs were inspected in 1999, 2000, and 2001. These programs are selected based on the lowest and highest success rates in the country as well as a random selection of programs of varying size that do not fall into these categories. Careful review and evaluation of the on-site validation program is ongoing under the validation committee of SART.

Funding for publication and validation has been committed by the CDC. Approximately $200,000 annually has been committed in the contract that SART has to collect and validate the data, At this time the funding covers primarily the validation program. The cost of collecting the data is almost entirely borne by SART and its member programs, and by extension their patients.

Both the CDC and SART have begun publishing results of clinical research based on the collected data. To ensure patient confidentiality, these data have been accorded the highest possible confidentiality status (known as 308D). Only the CDC and SART members have access to the data. For SART members to have such access, there are strict confidentiality and research requirements, the violation of some of which may result in civil and criminal penalties. Furthermore, all patients undergoing ART must agree to have their individual cycle data submitted through SART to the CDC.

Centers for Disease Control Model Program for Certification of Embryo Laboratories

In 1998 the CDC published their Proposed Model Program for the Certification of Embryo Laboratories as required by the FCSRCA. (10) This model program was implemented by publication in the *Federal Register* in 1998 and has been distributed to all states in the hope and expectation that the states can use it to draft their own requirements. California is one state that currently is considering further regulation of ART and is reviewing the model program to assist in development of its legislation. It is also expected that this model program will be used on a national level to help determine guidelines for oversight of ART.

Food and Drug Administration (FDA) Regulation of Reproductive Tissue

The FDA has recently proposed regulations that will affect ART. (11) The purpose of their proposal is "to establish a unified registration and product listing system for establishments that manufacture human cellular and tissue-based products." (11) It is expected that all ART clinics will be registered with the FDA beginning in 2003. The FDA is also concerned with qualification of donors, especially with respect to infectious disease testing and suitability of donor screening. They are also concerned with the handling, storage, and identification of reproductive tissue. The FDA's other areas of interest are product factors, including transmission of communicable disease, the processing of cells and tissue, clinical safety and effectiveness, promotion and labeling, and establishment of registration and product listing.

The FDA has received final comments regarding these regulations from ASRM and SART, as well as the American Association of Tissue Banks and the public. They have completed regulations requiring registration of ART establishments, and are in the final process of completing regulations regarding the determination of donor suitability, good tissue practices, and requirements for compliance and inspections. (12) Many of the comments received by the FDA have expressed concern over the potential impact of the proposed regulations on patient care, choice and cost, and duplication of oversight in ART laboratories.

Furthermore, the FDA has recently claimed authority over procedures involving transfer or potential transfer of genetic material in ART laboratories, including somatic cell nuclear transfer, cytoplasmic transfer, and coculture of embryos. The FDA is requiring submission and approval of an Investigational New Drug (IND) application prior to allowing such research. Therefore, somatic cell nuclear transfer, both reproductive and therapeutic, is prohibited unless such approval is given, and currently no such approvals have been given. Six ART programs performing cytoplasmic transfer on a research basis have received individual letters instructing them not to continue such research. The FDA has also stated that lymphocyte immune therapy for recurrent pregnancy loss cannot be performed unless there is submission and approval of an IND application. Implementation of these and other potential regulations could have far-reaching impact in ART programs, so professional organizations are currently evaluating these initiatives carefully and formulating a response.

New York State Task Force

The New York State Task Force on Life and The Law reported in April 1998 on assisted reproductive technologies and analysis, and made recommendations for public policy. (13) This task force was created by executive order in 1985 and charged with recommending policy on a host of issues raised by medical advances, including those in ART. For each issue the task force addresses, it recommends policy for the State of New York in the form of legislation, regulation, public education, or other measures. The recent report has raised considerable interest and public awareness about regulation of ART. The task force has received input from many professionals and the public concerning all aspects of ART, and will continue to refine its recommendations.

American Bar Association

The American Bar Association (ABA) Section of Family Law has a committee on laws of reproduction and genetic technology. In June 1998, this committee produced a working draft of a Model Assisted Reproductive Technologies Act. The National Conference of Commissioners on Uniform State Laws (NCUSL) proposed a Uniform Parentage Act (2000) to the ABA. This was rejected, but will be revised and resubmitted.

RESOLVE

RESOLVE is the national consumer organization dedicated to education, advocacy, and support of infertile people. RESOLVE's policy and public statements regarding oversight have been stated after careful consideration of their mission. (14) RESOLVE sees the basic principles for oversight as including quality medical care, quality assurance of laboratory facilities and clinical practice, protection from undue risks throughout the treatment process, education, counseling, informed consent, maintenance of choice of options for treatment, quality research, enforcement of provider noncompliance sanctions, and consumer/patient involvement in the process. RESOLVE believes that oversight should include areas such as the interests of both patients and the resulting children, standards of practice, oversight of embryo laboratories, mandatory reporting, validation of reporting, regulation of emerging experimental treatment, reproductive tissue screening, advertising and marketing controls, third-party concerns, and commercial interests.

RESOLVE's biggest area of concern and caution involves equal access to care, especially with respect to insurance coverage, while retaining flexibility in patient decision making. RESOLVE is committed to the development of evidence-based decision making for patients as well. RESOLVE also is concerned about the financial and insurance aspects of treatment, and is interested in protecting the patients from further expensive regulatory mechanisms. The organization is focused on the problem of the uneasiness, ambivalence, and lack of awareness by the public regarding reproductive medicine. In the United States, there are ongoing serious issues regarding restricting the availability and use of ART services. Since 1999, another consumer interest group, the American Infertility Association (AIA) has also advocated on behalf of infertile people.

Summary of Professional Initiatives to Increase Oversight of ART in the United States

It can be seen that there are numerous governmental, professional, and lay organizations working toward enhanced oversight of ART in the United States. Both SART and ASRM are cooperating with all of these organizations, including the CDC, congress, the FDA, FTC, and NIH, and other nongovernmental interested parties such as RESOLVE, the American Medical Association, the Centers for Medicare and Medicaid Services, the American Bar Association, the American College of Obstetricians and Gynecologists and the New York State Task Force. Indeed, it would be difficult to identify another area of medicine that has proposed and implemented so much self-regulation, and that has developed as many oversight relationships with government and other professional and lay organizations.

RECENT INITIATIVES BY SART TO INCREASE OVERSIGHT

In the last 3 years, SART has increased significantly its requirements for membership. To become and stay a member of SART, a clinic must report its results according to the FCSRCA, agree to on-site validation of reported success rates, and have laboratory accreditation that involves on-site laboratory inspection. In 1998, SART also made it a requirement for all medical directors of embryology laboratories to be Board-certified reproductive endocrinologists or active-status reproductive endocrinologists. Clinics must also adhere to the ethical, practice, laboratory, and advertising guidelines published by ASRM and SART. Membership can be, and has been, revoked for failure to comply with the above requirements.

On-site inspections of compliance with the SART guidelines were initiated in 2000 for randomly selected programs. Indeed, in the last year several programs have been instructed to modify their advertising and marketing practices to keep them in compliance with SART guidelines. A much more rigorous approach has also been taken to reporting deadlines and to identifying and reporting nonresponding clinics. As noted above, SART has also initiated a consultation program for clinics with low pregnancy rates so that they can be assisted in improving their success rates. As of 2002, participation in this program will be mandatory for clinics with pregnancy rates below statistically calculated standards, if clinics are to maintain their membership in

SART. Additionally, SART has expanded its membership to laboratory, nursing, and mental health professionals on an individual basis so that it can better represent all those involved in ART. Over 95% of United States IVF programs belong to SART.

PROPOSED OVERSIGHT OF ART IN THE UNITED STATES

National Coalition for Oversight of the Assisted Reproductive Technologies

In November 1995, the ASRM and SART joined in calling for an independent authority for oversight of ART programs and expressed a willingness to assist in development of such an oversight body. In 1997 SART established the National Coalition for Oversight of the Assisted Reproductive Technologies (NCOART) initially as a subcommittee of SART. In 1998 ASRM and SART participated in a national conference sponsored by the CDC, RESOLVE, and NABER: "Approaches to ART Oversight: What's Best in the U.S.?" (1) This conference brought together interested U.S. professionals, government experts, and consumers, as well as others from around the world, to discuss approaches to ART oversight in the United States.

The oversight committee had, as its initial mission statement, "to serve as an interdisciplinary advisory body that, on an ongoing basis, fosters quality assurance of ART services for the consumer, provider, and public at large by monitoring and evaluating reporting and use of ART success rates." Initial voting members of the oversight committee included SART with one clinical and one laboratory representative, ASRM, and RESOLVE. Liaison members are the CDC, FDA, FTC, and any other designated participatory governmental agency. Working group members include the American Association of Tissue Banks, (AATB), the ABA, and the American Infertility Association (AIA). Initially, the oversight committee functioned as a committee of SART. Subsequently the committee was renamed the National Coalition for Oversight of Assisted Reproductive Technologies (NCOART), with the chair of the committee rotating every two years between SART and RESOLVE. Each participating organization funds its own representatives' expenses, and SART underwrites the meeting expenses and provides administrative support. This committee meets twice annually and has made significant progress in identifying issues, making recommendations, and following up on issues.

The committee is not a regulatory body. Rather, it functions as a clearinghouse for issues and can make recommendations that can be implemented, if desired, by the individual organizations belonging to NCOART according to their own jurisdiction, deliberations, and conclusions. The goal of NCOART is to be a proactive agent for promoting systemic change:

1. To foster communication/dialogue about ART
2. To serve as a leader in identifying and examining issues in ART
3. To encourage appropriate groups to address areas of concern
4. To assist in review of outcomes to implement change intended to improve quality of care (15)

This review documents the significant regulation and oversight of ART procedures in the United States. However, there are many diverse overseeing authorities and organizations with the resultant numerous inconsistencies and omissions. Given this situation, NCOART is a forum for continuing discussion regarding provision of ART in the United States including the development of further regulation.

Questions and Answers Regarding ART Oversight in the United States

The models used in other countries, such as United Kingdom, Australia, France, and Canada, were extensively presented and reviewed at the February 1998 conference sponsored by the CDC, RESOLVE, and NABER. (1) Information gleaned from that meeting has been used by all organizations in their considerations of further development of oversight. At that conference several questions were asked regarding the best approaches to ART oversight in the United States. The answers to these questions have been used by SART in determining the course it will recommend for the future. These questions are addressed below.

The first question asked was "What are the critical gaps in approaches to ART oversight in the United States?" The answers were a lack of sanctions in the current system, problems with lack of funding for embryo research, incomplete and nonuniform documentation and reporting, inadequate quality assurance requirements, incomplete and nonuniform informed consent, lack of mandatory availability of counseling, lack of consumer input, inadequate donor screening and standards, lack of insurance, and lack of mandatory universal standards or a code of practice. It was felt, however, that these gaps could be rectified by initiatives in the United States. Indeed, many of these issues are in the process of being addressed by changes already completed or being considered in the regulatory process.

A second question asked was "How could new technical issues and new issues be addressed by additional oversight?" The answers included an oversight committee, SART research committee, local institutional review boards, national funding, nongovernmental committees, and improved guidelines for research innovations and standards of care.

Another concern, as always, was "How should the increased oversight be financed?" It was felt that a number of possibilities existed, including through insurance coverage, through a combination of public and private funding, or a combination of patients, infertility centers, and insurance and the public.

Another question was "Does the current system protect the consumers, and if not, what should be done?" It was generally concluded that the current approach to ART oversight in the United States is inadequate. Solutions require the mandatory availability of counseling, a mandatory code of practice, meaningful sanctions, improved information and informed consent for patients, mandatory laboratory oversight, mandatory record keeping and reporting, more consumer input, improved donor recruiting and screening standards, improved criteria for research, and improved insurance coverage.

Another concern raised was "Does the current system protect providers, and if not, what could be done?" It was also concluded that the current system had inadequate protection for providers and that it is important to identify a recognized body that can set standards, provide better coverage and cooperation from insurance companies, provide medical-legal protection for physicians practicing ART, better availability of research institutional review boards, and a code of practice to protect against unreasonable requests.

The question was asked, "Is there fair and equitable access to ART in the United States and if not, what were the barriers to access?" It was felt that there is not fair and equitable access because of individual financial constraints and insurance companies' failure to provide adequate coverage for ART, exacerbated by the lack of education and information regarding ART; lack of counseling especially with respect to moral, religious, and cultural views; misperceptions and uninformed social attitudes that are negative toward ART; media sensationalization of ART, both good and bad; state mandates; lack of oversight of vendors in the industry; the Employee Retirement Income Security Act (ERISA) which places limitations on health insurance liability for employers; nonaccommodating employers and provider attitudes; and geography, race, and quality of care.

Given the wide international experience in ART, the question was asked "Is there an international model or attributes of one that could be adopted in the United States?" It was concluded by all that the U.S. situation is unique, and that none of the international models are entirely adaptable to this country. However, in general, those at the meeting felt that accreditation was superior to licensing, that oversight should show a flexibility of language so that the oversight authority will not be unduly constrained as future unknown developments occur, and that there should be significant consumer participation. It was felt that legislation should be avoided when possible because of its tendency to restrict future choice, that consistency of documentation and publication should be striven for, and that adequate financing of ART is necessary.

Another question is "Are there are other forms of oversight in the United States that might be applied to ART?" Suggestions included UNOS, which oversees organ transplant in the United States, the FDA, the SART oversight committee, the New York State Cardiovascular Surgery Oversight, the Recombinant DNA National Committee, insurance companies, international standard-setting bodies, a registry for third-party donors, and the FTC. However, it was felt that none of these organizational models would be able to provide, by themselves, the appropriate oversight of ART in the United States.

Advantages and Disadvantages of Oversight

A great deal of experience has been gained in the United States by many professionals, government agencies, and other organizations regarding oversight of ART. It is not clear at this time what the final model in the United States will be, although some of the basic structures have been put in place, as described above. There are certain advantages and disadvantages of oversight, and it is hoped that as we move forward, we will be able to recognize these in developing the optimal system for the United States.

The advantages of oversight are that it establishes national standards, recognizes the uniqueness of ART, promotes high-quality patient care, ensures minimum standards of care, improves research, and protects patients' interests. Other advantages are that it provides a forum for national debate and participation, permits ethics statements that can be mandated by law, allows precedence in other fields to be used, increases society's confidence in and acceptance of ART, and potentially can increase insurance funding for ART.

Nevertheless, all oversight also carries with it disadvantages, as have been clearly recognized by practitioners from other countries, such as United Kingdom, France, Australia, and Canada. (1) Oversight requires funding and requires mechanisms of enforcement as well as the support of overseers, clinics, and patients. Oversight may fail to solve problems. It does not prevent psychopathic, sociopathic, or illegal behavior. It complicates legal issues of intent and due process, vis-a-vis criminal behavior versus inadvertent error in the practice of medicine. Furthermore, there is serious concern that oversight could interfere in the practice of medicine. This may be by intent, as with the current restrictions on embryo research, or may be unintentional, as with the Fertility Clinic Success Rate Certification Act whose clinic-specific success rate reporting requirements has caused some clinics to attempt to maximize their reported success rates by altering their practice of medicine. Oversight can also interfere in patients' rights; for example, AB-2209 in California required mandatory screening and places limitations on care based on a patient's history of infectious disease. Oversight can discriminate against some patients, increase costs to all patients, and politicize medical and personal issues.

The Hierarchy of Interest

Given this very complex situation of numerous interested government, professional, and lay organizations and individuals, and given the advantages and disadvantages of oversight, what is the best way to proceed? First, it is important to emphasize that SART and ASRM are committed to the concept of oversight of ART. We are, however, also committed to the concept of appropriate oversight and do not want the United States to implement an oversight program that is reactionary, ill conceived, and not suited to the best long-term interests of all the interested parties in the infertility industry. There are different parties involved in oversight, including patients, providers, and the public. The patients are represented by payers and RESOLVE, the public by the government, CDC, FDA, FTC, ABA, IRBs, and the NIH. Providers have numerous representatives including SART, ASRM, Society of Reproductive Endocrinologists (SRE), Reproductive Biologists Professional Group (RBPG), Mental Health Professional Group (MHPG), Nurses Professional Group (NPG), American College of Obstetricians and Gynecologists (ACOG), American Medical Association (AMA), College of American Pathologists (CAP), Reproductive Laboratories Technology Professional Group (RLTPG), American Association of Bioanalysts (AAB), and hospital, university, and industry groups, some of which are represented by the Biotechnology Industry Organization (BIO). There is considerable overlap of interest among all of these groups, and yet clearly each has its own constituency, mission, and interests (figure 1.1).

To develop a successful oversight authority in the United States, it is essential that a partnership of patients, providers, and the public be developed. Such oversight needs to be independent from any one interested party and have the authority for mandatory enforcement. It is critical that any mandates be flexible enough to accommodate rapid changes in technology, medical needs, and social perspectives. Standards of care need to be set and a few specific regulations developed. Oversight should be financed by all three interested parties, while avoiding polarizing political and moral agendas.

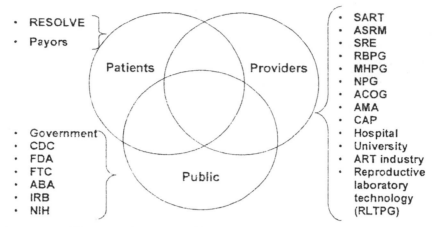

Figure 1.1   Different Parties Interested in Oversight of ART
Source: Adamson. Regulation of ART in the U.S. *Fertil Steril* 2002.

Current proposals for mandates for an oversight authority that are supported by SART include mandatory compliance, meaningful sanctions, uniformity in reporting, on-site inspection and validation, and development of practice standards, research standards, education standards, and counseling standards, as well as access to insurance coverage and research funding, and a limitation of regulation. Once established, any oversight authority must establish its own priorities: are they to meet consumer needs, allay public fears, protect embryos and future children, or control physicians and research? SART and others will continue to evaluate, discuss, and make proposals for government, professional, and public consideration.

In all of these considerations, the hierarchy of interest should be taken into account (figure 1.2). Simply stated, this means that those who have the greatest interest in the outcomes of ART should have the greatest influence in the oversight authority. At the top of the hierarchy of interest are the patients, and with them their gametic material and future children. In all discussions and consideration, focus should be on providing the highest possible quality and value care for this group. Interests and considerations of others involved in ART should be secondary. It can be argued that physicians, embryologists, and other scientists who have developed this industry, who currently provide care and will provide the research and new technology of the future, have the secondary level of interest, as it is their primary focus professionally in life. Their interests should be second only to those of the patients. Third in the hierarchy of interest come professional organizations involved in ART such as SART, ASRM, RESOLVE, embryologists' organizations, nurses, and mental health professionals. They also have a large and focused commitment to this field.

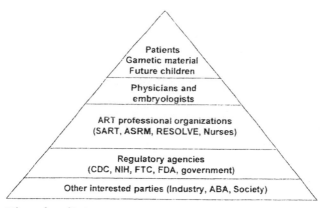

Figure 1.2   Hierarchy of Interest
Source: Adamson. Regulation of ART in the U.S. *Fertil Steril* 2002.

Fourth, regulatory agencies, such as the CDC, FTC, FDA, NIH, and other federal agencies, have an important role to play in the development of oversight. However, ART is only a small area of their interest and expertise, and generally their control over the industry should be more limited than those higher in the hierarchy of interest. Finally, there are obviously other interested parties representing society. These include groups such as the ABA, industry organizations, and the general public. Their input to oversight is extremely important, but the values and mission of those who do not have a direct interest in the outcome of ART should carry less influence in the final development of oversight than those higher in the hierarchy of interest who are much more directly affected. Nevertheless, society has an overriding interest in some aspects of reproductive technology, such as reproductive somatic cell nuclear transfer, where it is legitimate for legislation to set the social and legal standards.

CONCLUSION

In conclusion, significant progress has been made in the United States in developing oversight. Reproductive technology is a complex and rapidly changing clinical, scientific, and ethical field of human endeavor. It involves highly visible and emotional issues. We live in a heterogeneous society in which there is a multiplicity of views on each and every issue. We will be successful in the United States only by ensuring that all those with an interest in oversight have a meaningful role in its development. It is important that the hierarchy of interest be taken into account, allowing those with the greatest stake in ART to help develop oversight which thus ensures the maximum rewards to those most affected by infertility and other reproductive issues.

NOTES

1. Approaches to ART oversight: what's best in the U.S.? Washington, D.C.: Centers for Disease Control Conference Summary, 12–13 February 1998.

2. The Fertility Clinic Success Rate and Certification Act of 1992 (Public Law 102–493).

3. Rules and Regulations of the State of New York, Part 52 of Title 10 (Health). Tissue Banks and Non-transplant Anatomic Banks. Albany, New York: State of New York Department of Health, 1992.

4. California Health and Safety Code. Division 2, Chapter 4.1: Tissue Banks. Berkeley, CA: State of California, Department of Health Services, 1992.

5. The College of American Pathologists/American Society for Reproductive Medicine Reproductive laboratory accreditation program. Northfield, IL: College of American Pathologists, 1996.

6. American Society for Reproductive Medicine and Society for Assisted Reproductive Technology. Birmingham, AL.

7. American College of Obstetricians and Gynecologists. Washington, DC.

8. Chapko KM, Weaver MR, Chapko MK, Pasta D, Adamson GD. Stability of in vitro fertilization-embryo transfer success rates from the 1989, 1990, and 1991 clinic-specific outcome assessments. *Fertil Steril* 1995;64:757–63.

9. Centers for Disease Control and Prevention. Reporting pregnancy success rates from assisted reproductive technology programs. 62CFR 45259, 26 August 1997.

10. Implementation of the Fertility Clinic Success Rate and Certification Act of 1992: Proposed model program for the certification of embryo laboratories; notice. Federal Register 63(215); 6 November 1998 (60178–60189).

11. Establishment registration and listing for manufacturers of human cellular and tissue-based products. Federal Register 63(93); 14 May 1998 (26744-26755).

12. The American Association of Tissue Banks standards for tissue banking. McLean, VA: American Association of Tissue Banks, 1996.

13. Assisted reproductive technologies analysis and recommendations for public policy. New York: The New York State Task Force on Life and the Law, April 1998.

14. Oversight of the assisted reproductive technologies. Somerville, MA: RESOLVE, Presented at: Approaches to ART oversight: What's best in the U.S.? Washington, D.C.: Centers for Disease Control Conference Summary, February 12–13, 1998.

15. The Goal of NCOART. NCOART Minutes, 26 October 1998.

2

Progress We Can Be Proud Of: U.S. Trends in Assisted Reproduction over the First 20 Years

James P. Toner

Louise Brown was born July 25, 1978, after years of diligent work on in vitro fertilization by the pioneering British team of Robert Edwards and Patrick Steptoe. (1) Scientists and clinicians around the world understood the significance of this event, and clamored to reproduce it. In the United States, several teams undertook the challenge, and Drs. Howard and Georgeanna Jones were the first to be rewarded for their efforts with the birth of Elizabeth Carr on December 28, 1981. (2) Success by other U.S. teams soon followed.

The dramatic expansion of in vitro fertilization (IVF) around the world, and the allied therapies of embryo cryopreservation, donor egg, GIFT, zygote intrafallopian transfer (ZIFT), and intracytoplasmic sperm injection (ICSI) as well, testifies to the commitment of innumerable clinicians and scientists to assist infertile couples with their hope for healthy children.

In the United States, efforts to catalogue IVF activity began in 1985, and have continued ever since. This reporting was entirely voluntary, but participation was high. The special interest group within the ASRM, now called SART, has coordinated this annual tabulation since its first publication in 1988. In 1992, reporting became federally mandated with the passage of the Fertility Clinic Success Rate and Certification Act. (3) The first publication stemming from this law tabulated ART cycles performed in 1995.

MATERIALS AND METHODS

Beginning in 1988, reports have been published in *Fertility and Sterility* that tabulate the clinical ART activity in the United States from 1985 through 1999, the last available annual report. (4–17) These reports are the source of the results reported here.

The reports on activity from 1985 through 1990 were based on data collected by Medical Research International on instruction from the special interest group for IVF within the then AFS. This reporting required cycle-specific information and was deemed cumbersome. For the 1987 report and thereafter, this special interest group acquired the name of the Society for Assisted Reproductive Technology, and its Registry Committee has been responsible for this effort.

The reports for the activity in 1991 through 1993 were managed directly by the Registry Committee through simplified "Summary Sheets," which captured some general outcome data but no cycle-specific information.

The report for 1994 cycles was based on data collected under a contract with a national accounting firm (KPMG). This process collected cycle-specific information, but was extremely time-consuming for the clinics, expensive for the AFS, unwieldy for the Registry Committee, and consequently untenable for future collections.

Since 1995, the Registry Committee has collected data via its own Clinical Outcome Reporting System (CORS). This computer program was developed to collect the minimum cycle-specific information judged to be needed by the SART, ASRM, and the Centers for Disease Control and Prevention (CDC), which by that time had been given a mandate to report on national and clinic-specific outcomes. The CORS has been revised since to reflect evolving clinical practice.

Because the method of collecting data, and clinical practice itself have changed over time, the annual reports contain some changes that are pertinent when interpreting trends in practice and outcome.

1. Standard IVF, GIFT, donor egg, and transfers using cryopreserved embryos were first reported in the 1985 report. The first published report of GIFT appeared in 1984. (18) The 1988 report first reported ZIFT, although the practice was first described in 1986. (19) Transfers of cryopreserved embryos derived from donor eggs, host cycles, and combination cycles were first reported in 1991. Research cycles and embryo banking were first specified in 1996.

2. Micromanipulation of eggs to improve fertilization was first reported in 1992. The first techniques were reported about 1990—partial zona dissection in 1989 (20) and subzonal insertion in 1990 (21)—but neither proved particularly effective. A more effective form of micromanipulation, ICSI, was first described in 1988, (22) but was not shown to be highly effective until 1992. (23) It was singled out in the 1995 report, at which time other forms of micromanipulation were dropped.

3. Multiple pregnancy rates (per delivery) were not reported for the activity in 1985 and 1986, but have been reported since.

4. The importance of female age has been known from early on, but the reports have divided the data by different female ages, as our understanding of this dimension has improved. From 1988 to 1990, female age was reported as <25, 25 to 29, 30 to 34, 35 to 39, and 40+ years. The years 1991 to 1994 divided age only into two categories: <40 and 40+ years. In 1995 and 1996, three categories were used: <35, 35 to 39, and 40+ years. In 1997 and 1998, four categories were reported: <35, 35 to 37, 38 to 40, and 41+ years. In 1999, five categories were used: <35, 35 to 37, 38 to 40, 41 to 42, 43+ years.
5. Cycles from programs in Canada were included from 1991 through 1995, but not before or since.
6. Aggregate clinical activity in the United States between 1981 and 1984 is not reported in any collected form.

RESULTS

Outcomes of 647,208 cycles of treatment, covering activity during the years 1985 through 1999, have been reported to the registry. Among these, 155,661 clinical pregnancies occurred, which led to 128,608 births and the delivery of 177,745 infants.

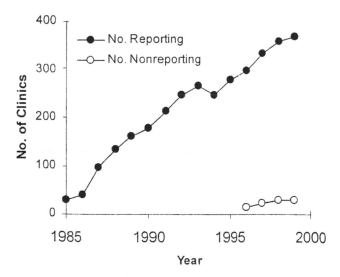

Figure 2.1   Number of Clinics Reporting Data to the National Registry for Each Reporting Year. Since 1996, the CDC has also published the number of U.S. ART clinics known not to have reported their cases.
Source: Toner. ART trends in the U.S. *Fertil Steril* 2002.

The number of clinics (Fig. 2.1), cycles, and babies born (Fig. 2.2) has steadily increased over the years. About 400 clinics in the United States were operating in 1999; only a minority fails to report results (approximately 10%). Most of the nonreporting clinics are not thought to be large volume clinics, so most of the activity is captured in those that report. In parallel with the number of clinics has been a steady increase in the number of cycles of therapy and deliveries: in 1999, almost 90,000 cycles were performed and more than 20,000 deliveries were reported. In contrast, in 1981 only one delivery occurred in the United States by these methods.

Tubal transfer procedures (GIFT and ZIFT) were introduced in the mid-1980s, and were soon thereafter being tracked in the national database. These procedures were recommended as more physiological, because in normal reproduction early embryos are found in the tubes, not the uterus. Early results were encouraging, and the registry data showed higher success with both GIFT and ZIFT over standard IVF year after year, until about 1995. No randomized controlled studies confirmed the superiority of these tubal transfer methods, (24) and they were more invasive and expensive than standard IVF. Examination of these trends suggests that the success rates of GIFT and ZIFT reached a plateau at about 35% to 40% in 1992. At that time, IVF success was only about 25%. However, IVF success rates have continued to climb, and now equal those achieved in GIFT and ZIFT. At their peak in the late 1980s and early 1990s, GIFT and ZIFT cycles accounted for more than 25% of all fresh stimulated cy-

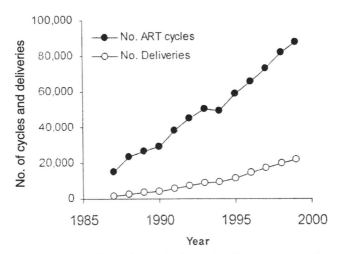

Figure 2.2   The Number of Total ART Cycles and Deliveries Reported to the National Registry. Steady increases in both are noted.
Source: Toner. ART trends in the U.S. *Fertil Steril* 2002.

cles. As the difference in success became smaller, their use declined dramatically (Fig 2.3). Currently, <3% of stimulated cycles employ tubal transfer.

Success rates were initially low for cases with male factor infertility due to
low fertilization rates, and led to the separate reporting of cycles with and
without male factor infertility. In the early 1990s, cycles with male factor infertility were both less likely to fertilize (20% to 30% less), and less likely to
deliver (about 15%) even with a successful embryo transfer. Micromanipulative procedures of the egg were developed and introduced in the late 1980s to
remedy this situation. Initially, efforts were focused on the zona pellucida. In
partial zona dissection, the zona was cut in hopes that sperm would be able to
enter through the slit. In sub-zonal insertion (or insemination), a few sperm
were placed in the perivitelline space, between the zona and egg, using a
pipette. Success with these approaches was limited, but many clinics began to
employ them because the prognosis for severe male factor infertility was so
poor otherwise. The registry began to collect information on these procedures
in 1992 (Fig. 2.4). In that same year, the initial report on ICSI was published.
Over the next few years, its superiority and effectiveness became readily apparent. By 1995, the majority of clinics were offering ICSI for male factor infertility treatments, and the registry began to collect only the number of ICSI
cycles. As ICSI became routine, the difference in fertilization and overall success rates between "male factor" and all other cases became smaller, and has

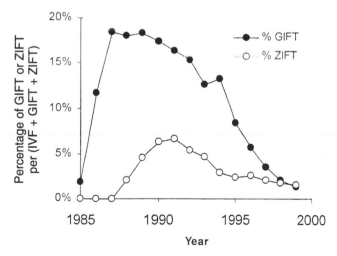

**Figure 2.3   GIFT gained popularity quickly but has become less common in recent
years. ZIFT, introduced later, has never been as popular and has also become less common.**
Source: Toner. ART trends in the U.S. *Fertil Steril* 2002.

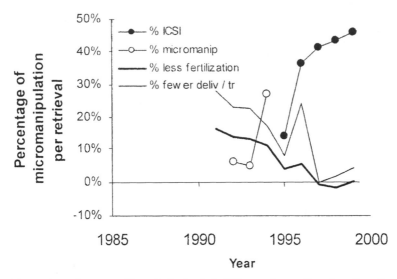

Figure 2.4 Success with male factor infertility was lower than for other diagnoses. Cycles with male factor infertility were less likely to achieve fertilization (initially as high as 30% less) and delivery, even with an embryo transfer (initially 15% lower). Consequently, micromanipulative techniques were used in an effort to increase fertilization in cases of abnormal semen. Early efforts using subzonal insertion and partial zona disection (% micromanipulation) were quickly replaced by the more effective ICSI (% ICSI). From 1992 through 1994, these techniques were not distinguished within the report. Since 1995, only ICSI has been reported. The "% less fertilization" and "% fewer deliveries per transfer" were calculated by dividing the difference in rates between cycles with and without male factor infertility by the rate for cycles without male factor infertility in the youngest reported age bracket (1988–1989: all women; 1990–1995: women < 40 years old; 1995–1999: women < 35 years old).
Source: Toner. ART trends in the U.S. *Fertil Steril* 2002.

essentially vanished since about 1997. In 1999, more than 45% of all cycles employed ICSI as a component of the therapy.

Overall pregnancy and delivery rates have been steadily increasing for all types of ART treatment (Fig. 2.5). In the most recent years, donor eggs have been substantially the most successful therapy, whereas the earlier differences among IVF, GIFT, and ZIFT have vanished (and all remain less effective than donor eggs). Success with cryopreserved embryos has always been lowest of the major therapies. Pregnancy rates per transfer for IVF were only about 15% in the early reporting years, but have now risen to nearly 40%. Similarly, donor egg therapy has risen from a 25% pregnancy per transfer rate to 50%. Even cryopreservation cycles, have shown dramatic improvement over time: before 1990, the success rate was about 10% per transfer; now it is more than 20%. As mentioned above, GIFT and ZIFT rates were initially

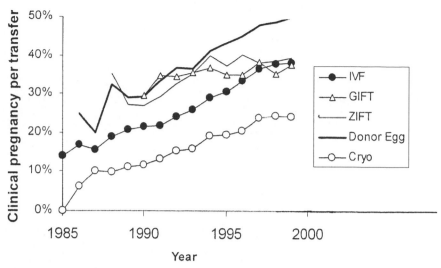

Figure 2.5 The clinical pregnancy rate per transfer has steadily increased over the term of the registry reports. These increases were seen in all types of ART. The higher success rates of GIFT and ZIFT in early years have vanished, which may explain their less frequent use. Donor egg therapy is the most effective common therapy, and cryopreservation the least.
Source: Toner. ART trends in the U.S. *Fertil Steril* 2002.

higher than IVF rates overall, but have held steady at about 35% to 40% for the past 8 years. This may reflect the gametes and/or embryos spending much less time in the embryology laboratory with these tubal transfer methods than with the other techniques, so there is potentially less to improve.

Pregnancy loss rates declined across major therapies until about 1990, when they plateaued between 15% and 20% per clinical pregnancy (figure 2.6). In the earliest reporting years, loss rates were above 40% for IVF but are now less than 20%. Even donor egg therapy, which generally has had the lowest pregnancy loss rates (currently about 15%), had loss rates almost twice as high in the earlier years. The loss rates for cryopreserved embryos and GIFT tend to be higher than with other therapies, approximating 25% in recent years.

Multiple pregnancy rates (per deliver) have shown a slight increase over the years, until recently when they have begun to decline (figure 2.7). These rates are strongly influenced by the therapy rendered: they are lowest among those using cryopreserved embryos (just above 25% in recent years), and highest when using donor eggs (above 40%). The multiple pregnancy rates have hovered in the middle 30% range for IVF, GIFT, and ZIFT in the past decade.

Concern about these rates led practitioners to reduce the number of embryos transferred, resulting in dramatic declines in the rates of triplet, and especially

James P. Toner

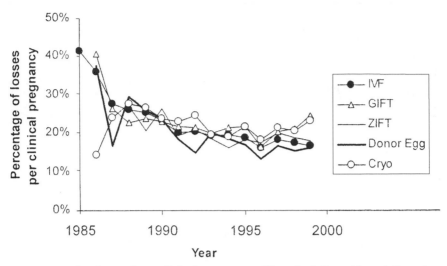

Figure 2.6   The chance that a clinical pregnancy will not be followed by a delivery has held steady at about 20% over the years for all therapies. The highest rates of failure are seen amongst cryopreserved embryo transfer cycles, and the lowest among donor egg cycles.
Source: Toner. ART trends in the U.S. *Fertil Steril* 2002.

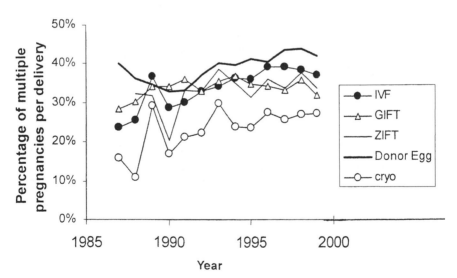

Figure 2.7   Multiple Pregnancy Rates Are Illustrated for the Major ART Therapies over the Years of Reporting to the Registry. Gradual increases in these rates have been reversed in the most recent reporting years. These rates have been highest for donor egg therapy, lowest for cryopreserved embryo transfers, and intermediate for the other therapies.
Source: Toner. ART trends in the U.S. *Fertil Steril* 2002.

quadruplet, deliveries (figure 2.8). Because the reports only tabulate the rates of multiple pregnancy per delivery (rather than per clinical pregnancy), the reported rates include both the incidence of multiple pregnancies per clinical pregnancy, and the effect of any subsequent pregnancy losses (spontaneous or elective). Consequently, the reported declines might be due to lower rates of multiple pregnancy per se, or higher rates of pregnancy loss, or both, and it is not possible to assign relative proportions via the registry reports. It is noteworthy that the declines in the multiple pregnancy rate began before new guide-

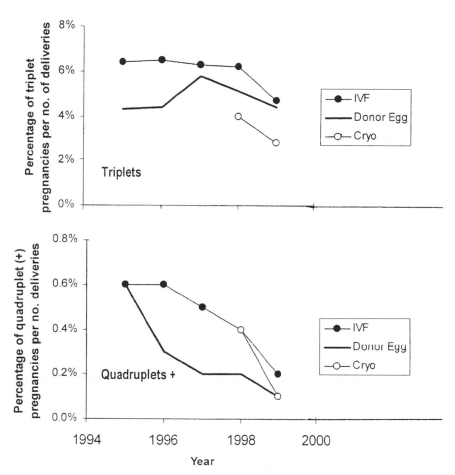

Figure 2.8 Examination of the "high-order" multiple pregnancy rates in the major therapies reveals declines since 1997 for triplets, and earlier for quadruplets and more. Moreover, the reduction in quadruplets and more has been quite dramatic: from 0.6% of deliveries, to no more than 0.2% in 1999. Rates for cryopreserved cycles were not reported until 1998.

Source: Toner. ART trends in the U.S. *Fertil Steril* 2002.

lines were issued (November 1999; 25) and in the complete absence of regulation. Whether further reductions will occur as the guidelines become adopted
will only become apparent with the publication of future registry reports.

The effect of the woman's age on success was recognized as important
early on. Reporting by age began with the 1988 cycles, and has been modi-
fied several times in the registry reports. Examination of success rates by age
clearly demonstrates not only the effect of age, but also the higher success
rates within age over time (Fig. 2.9). As women under age 35 do quite well

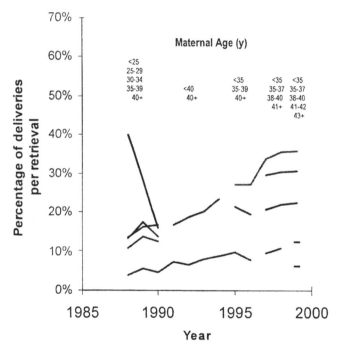

**Figure 2.9   The effect of maternal age on ART success has been known since the early
days of ART therapy. The registry reports have presented this effect in different age
brackets over the years (the key inset into the figure indicates the age brackets used during each reporting year). Lines are discontinuous when new age brackets were introduced, and continuous when the same age bracket was used in the new reporting year.
IVF success rates are illustrated; note the important effect of maternal age in all reporting years, and the gradual increase in success within each age bracket over time.
Lastly, note the evolution of the recognition that the major effect of age begins past age
35: in early reporting, three age brackets below age 35 were reported; now only one is.
Alternatively, the two brackets above age 35 have now become four distinct brackets,
each with objectively different prospects for ART success. The particularly high success
in the youngest women in 1988 appears to be anomalous.**
Source: Toner. ART trends in the U.S. *Fertil Steril* 2002.

in IVF, the bottom age brackets were combined; fertility declines rapidly as age 40 approaches, so the two age brackets above age 35 have become four.

DISCUSSION

The first 20 years of ART in the United States has brought remarkable improvements.

Introduction of New Therapies

Initially designed for couples in which the woman had irreparable tubal damage, ART has been extended to women with poor or no eggs (donor egg therapy), women with irreparable or absent uteri (host or surrogate uterus programs), women with embryos in excess of those to be replaced fresh (embryo cryopreservation), and men with serious sperm deficiencies (ICSI).

HIGHER SUCCESS FOR MAJOR THERAPIES

Pregnancy and delivery rates have persistently increased since the first reports. For example, IVF delivery rates per transfer have tripled, from about 10% to 30%. Donor egg delivery rates have doubled, from about 20% to above 40%. Even cryopreservation has improved: initial delivery rates of just over 10% per transfer are now over 20%, a doubling.

Streamlining of Treatments

In the early days of IVF, placing eggs or embryos directly into the tubes (GIFT or ZIFT) was both theoretically and factually more successful than routine IVF with intrauterine embryo transfer. Unfortunately, GIFT and ZIFT required a surgical transfer, with its attendant additional expense and discomfort. As routine IVF success became equal to GIFT and ZIFT, it became possible to forego these more complex and expensive treatments. Appropriately, practitioners have largely abandoned these therapies for the majority of patients.

REDUCED INCIDENCE OF MULTIPLE DELIVERIES

ART practitioners have long known that multiple pregnancies bring significant maternal and especially fetal risks. Many practitioners found their initial efforts to reduce high-order multiples by transferring fewer embryos were stymied by concurrent improvements in IVF (manifested by higher implantation rates). However, with the appropriate adjustment in the number of embryos to be transferred, the rate of multiple deliveries in excess of twins, has begun to drop. Triplets following IVF have dropped by a third (from about 6.5% to 4.5% in 1999), and in cryopreserved cycles by almost half (from 4% to about 2.5%). Deliveries of four or more infants have become quite rare: in IVF, 0.6% has become 0.2% in 1999; with donor eggs, 0.6% has become 0.1%, and with cryopreserved embryos, 0.4% in 1998 has become 0.1% in 1999. Given that the revised guidelines for the number of embryos to transfer was issued in late 1999, one might anticipate even further reductions in the 2000 dataset.

Favorable Results When Compared to Europe

When compared to the only other large and contemporaneous ART registry, which covers Europe and is maintained by ESHRE, (26) significant differences in outcomes are apparent. In the United States, pregnancy rates with all major therapies are substantially higher than in Europe, but so too are multiple pregnancy rates. For example, the clinical pregnancy rate per transfer for IVF in Europe for 1998 was 27.0% versus 37.8% in the United States. For donor egg treatments, 39.6% of European transfers led to clinical pregnancy, as compared to 48.7% in the United States. Even transfers of cryopreserved embryos were more often successful in the United States: 24.3% in the United States versus 14.5% in Europe. Although there was country to country variability in success within Europe, no country that did more than 500 cycles had a higher success rate than the United States in IVF, donor egg, or cryopreserved embryo transfers.

However, counterbalancing the higher pregnancy rates are higher multiple pregnancy rates. In Europe in 1998, IVF produced deliveries of twins in 23.9% of deliveries, triplets in 2.3%, and quadruplets (or more) in 0.1%. In the United States, the comparable rates were 31.7%, 6.2%, and 0.2%. These higher rates are problematic, but it is noteworthy that the multiple pregnancy rates in the United States declined in 1999 without an associated decline in overall pregnancy or delivery rates.

These improvements in success rates have been steady and persistent, and are testaments to the work of numerous investigators, the ready adoption of new methods by practitioners striving to give their patients every advantage, and the absence of legal impediments to changes in clinical practice. Recent FDA statements requiring that clinicians obtain federal approval (via the IND process) to offer cytoplasmic transfer, nuclear transfer, and embryo co-culture may herald the end of this rapid progress in our field. Nonetheless, the progress to date has been laudable, and investigators will no doubt continue to strive to provide their patients with the care they require, despite any obstacles.

NOTES

1. Edwards RG, Steptoe PC, Purdy JM. Clinical aspects of pregnancies established with cleaving embryos grown in vitro. *Br J Obstet Gynaecol* 1980;87:757–68.

2. Jones HW Jr, Jones GS, Andrews MC, Acosta A, Bundren C, Garcia, J, et al. The program for in vitro at Norfolk. *Fertil Steril* 1982;38:14–21.

3. Fertility Clinic Success Rate and Certification Act of 1992. (Public Law No. 102–493, 42 USC 263a-1 et seq.). Washington, DC: U.S. Congress, October 24, 1992.

4. Medical Research International and the American Fertility Society Special Interest Group. In vitro fertilization/embryo transfer in the United States: 1985 and 1986 results from the National IVF/ET Registry. *Fertil Steril* 1988;49:212–5.

5. Medical Research International and the Society of Assisted Reproductive Technology, the American Fertility Society. In vitro fertilization/embryo transfer in the United States: 1987 results from the National IVF-ET Registry. *Fertil Steril* 1989;51:13–9.

6. Medical Research International and the Society for Assisted Reproductive Technology, the American Fertility Society. In vitro fertilization-embryo transfer in the United States: 1988 results from the IVF-ET Registry. *Fertil Steril* 1990;53:13–20.

7. Medical Research International, Society for Assisted Reproductive Technology, the American Fertility Society. In vitro fertilization-embryo transfer (IVF-ET) in the United States: 1989 results from the IVF-ET Registry. *Fertil Steril* 1991;55:14–23.

8. Medical Research International, Society for Assisted Reproductive Technology (SART), the American Fertility Society. In vitro fertilization-embryo transfer (IVF-ET) in the United States: 1990 results from the IVF-ET Registry. *Fertil Steril* 1992;57:15–24.

9. Society for Assisted Reproductive Technology, the American Fertility Society. Assisted reproductive technology in the United States and Canada: 1991 results from the Society for Assisted Reproductive Technology generated from the American Fertility Society Registry. *Fertil Steril* 1993;59:956–62.

10. The American Fertility Society, Society for Assisted Reproductive Technology. Assisted reproductive technology in the United States and Canada: 1992 results generated from the American Fertility Society/Society for Assisted Reproductive Technology Registry. *Fertil Steril* 1994;62:1121–8.

11. Society for Assisted Reproductive Technology, American Society for Reproductive Medicine. Assisted reproductive technology in the United States and Canada: 1993 results generated from the American Society for Reproductive Medicine/Society for Assisted Reproductive Technology Registry. *Fertil Steril* 1995;64:13–21.

12. Society for Assisted Reproductive Technology, American Society for Reproductive Medicine. Assisted reproductive technology in the United States and Canada: 1994 results generated from the American Society for Reproductive Medicine/Society for Assisted Reproductive Technology Registry. *Fertil Steril* 1996;66:697–705.

13. Society for Assisted Reproductive Technology, the American Society for Reproductive Medicine. Assisted reproductive technology in the United States and Canada: 1995 results generated from the American Society for Reproductive Medicine/ Society for Assisted Reproductive Technology Registry. *Fertil Steril* 1998;69:389–98.

14. Society for Assisted Reproductive Technology, the American Society for Reproductive Medicine. Assisted reproductive technology in the United States: 1996 results generated from the American Society for Reproductive Medicine/Society for Assisted Reproductive Technology Registry. *Fertil Steril* 1999;71:798–807.

15. Society for Assisted Reproductive Technology, American Society for Reproductive Medicine. Assisted reproductive technology in the United States: 1997 results generated from the American Society for Reproductive Medicine/Society for Assisted Reproductive Technology Registry. *Fertil Steril* 2000;74:641–53.

16. Society for Assisted Reproductive Technology, American Society for Reproductive Medicine. Assisted reproductive technology in the United States: 1998 results generated from the American Society for Reproductive Medicine/Society for Assisted Reproductive Technology Registry. *Fertil Steril* 2002;77:18–31.

17. Society for Assisted Reproductive Technology, American Society for Reproductive Medicine. Assisted reproductive technology in the United States: 1999 results generated from the American Society for Reproductive Medicine/Society for Assisted Reproductive Technology Registry. *Fertil Steril* 2002;78:918–31.

18. Asch RH, Ellsworth LR, Balmaceda JP, Wong PC. Pregnancy after translaparoscopic gamete intrafallopian transfer. *Lancet* 1984;2:1034.

19. Devroey P, Braeckmans P, Smitz J, van Waesberghe L, Wisanto A, van Steirteghem A, Heytens L, Camus M. Pregnancy after translaproscopic zygote intrafallopian transfer on a patient with sperm antibodies, *Lancet* 1986;1:1329.

20. Malter HE, Cohen J. Partial zona dissection of the human oocyte: a nontraumatic method using micromanipulation to assist zona pellucida penetration. *Fertil Steril* 1989;51:139.

21. Fishel S, Jackson P, Antinori S, Johnson J, Grossi S, Versaci C. Subzonal insemination for the alleviation of infertility. *Fertil Steril* 1990;54:828.

22. Lanzendorf S, Maloney M, Ackerman S, Acosta A, Hodgen G. Fertilizing potential of acrosome-defective sperm following microsurgical injection into eggs. *Gamete Res* 1988;19:329–37.

23. Palermo G, Joris H, Devroey P, van Steirteghem AC. Pregnancies after intracytoplasmic injection of single spermatozoon into an oocyte. *Lancet* 1992;340:17–8.

24. Habana AE, Palter SF. Is tubal embryo transfer of any value? A meta-analysis and comparison with the Society for Assisted Reproductive Technology database. *Fertil Steril* 2001; 76:286–93.

25. American Society for Reproductive Medicine. *Guidelines on number of embryos transferred*. Birmingham, Alabama: American Society for Reproductive Medicine, 1999.

26. Nygren KG, Anderson AN. Assisted reproductive technology in Europe, 1998. results generated from European registers by ESHRE. *Hum Reprod* 2001; 16:2459–71.

3

Reproductive Technologies: Ethical and Religious Issues

Thomas A. Shannon

This article will discuss several ethical dimensions of assisted reproduction. First, I will identify general ethical issues that have not been fully evaluated, primarily because of the way the field of assisted reproduction developed. Second, I will argue that while Roman Catholicism has a fairly developed and clear teaching about assisted reproduction and that while some of this teaching has a value beyond the boundaries of this religion, ultimately the teaching lacks credibility because of use of a problematic understanding of natural law. The teaching is overly physicalist or biological in its development of norms, and this narrowness of interpretation impedes Catholicism from responding constructively to historical changes in marriage and in the family. Finally, I will develop aspects of Roman Catholic social ethics that could contribute to a discussion of assisted reproduction, particularly within the discussion of health insurance. Here I will be moving beyond a traditional understanding of natural law but will remain within the general context of Roman Catholic social teaching. While criticizing many aspects of traditional Roman Catholic teaching, I want to argue that there are, nonetheless, resources within this tradition that are both constructive and useful in evaluating this important, developing branch of reproductive medicine.

ASSISTED REPRODUCTION: AN OVERVIEW

The birth of Louise Brown in England in 1978 was a reproductive revolution as profound as the introduction of artificial contraceptives in the 1950s. For several years, Steptoe and Edwards had been doing animal experiments on *in vitro* fertilization with varying degrees of success. However, the main lines of the technique were established, and the outcome seemed to depend as much on luck as technique. Everything came together, though, in the birth of Louise Brown, and reproduction was never the same.

After this beginning, the use of this technology spread rapidly, first in England, Australia, and the United States and now around the world. Although it was far from established as successful, the technology moved immediately to the clinic. In the early decades of AR, few data were collected and few, if any, controlled studies were performed. Thus the details of AR were learned and gathered in a rather random fashion, remaining primarily within the particular clinic, since increased success gave the clinic a financial advantage. Fortunately, the technology itself and the various means of manipulating sperm, egg, and preimplantation embryo do not appear to be harmful to these entities. Nor does the technology appear to cause harm to the children born of the technology. The critical issue, though, is that we have learned this from clinical practice, not from carefully designed research protocols.

Because of the rapid move from experimental procedure to clinical practice, few, if any, regulatory standards were in place. There were no requirements for any type of board certification or for any particular training in human reproduction or obstetrics, with the possible exception of assisting at the birth itself. (Midwives, for example, need certification by the state, as well as those in the field of ob/gyn before they call assist at birth.) The same was true of the clinics themselves. These were essentially private enterprises and were not regulated either by the state or the medical establishment. Who was entitled to do what and based on what training and credentials was simply unclear. The alleged training standard of "see one, do one, teach one" appeared to be normative, not stereotypical.

As attention focused on the growing field and as the practice spread more widely, a core procedure of egg retrieval, fertilization, incubation, and implantation became established. This was helped by the publication of articles in professional journals, the establishment of several journals devoted to AR, new training programs at medical schools, and the development of guidelines by professional medical societies. More attention thus was paid to the biology of reproduction and the technologies used to assist in reproduction. Now, almost twenty years after Louise Brown's birth, AR is an accepted part of standard medical practice, some dimensions of which are now covered by many insurance plans.

But critical issues still remain. While AR is widely available in both hospitals and private clinics, access to it is still restricted, primarily by costs, with fees for a single IVF cycle ranging from $8,000 to $10,000. Although AR is covered by some insurance plans, what the plans cover varies widely. Some will pay for infertility workups; others will also pay for one or two cycles of in vitro fertilization. Still other plans will pay for some procedures and not others. Even if insurance pays for some parts of the procedure, there will be many out-of-pocket expenses, such as travel costs, hotel stays, and time off from work. And while costs are coming down, prices vary dramatically from clinic to clinic. Hardly anyone becomes pregnant on the first cycle, so cycles will be repeated and often new technologies used. One is quickly beyond one's insurance coverage. Thus accessibility to the technology is limited both by insurance limits and one's disposable income.

Some clinics pro-rate the costs of IVF, refunding many costs if no child is born. For example, Pacific Fertility Center, with branches in Los Angeles, San Francisco, and Sacramento, recently took out a half page ad in the *New York Times*. (1) For a set fee, the client receives a single cycle of IVF with either her eggs or a donor's eggs and, if she does not get pregnant on this try, will have all the remaining frozen embryos implanted. If the client does not carry a pregnancy for at least twelve weeks, she receives a 90% refund. Pacific Fertility Center also offers a variety of other financial options: a single cycle for customary fees, shared IVF egg donor programs so that two couples can split the fees, a plan for women forty-three years of age and younger that allows up to three IVF cycles for a single fee, and discounts of up to 35% for couples demonstrating financial need. There is also a *pro bono* grant program that provides free IVF services. (2)

A 1983 study, focusing on the first five years of IVF programs in Britain, Australia, and the United States, showed that while success rates of various AR technologies were increasing, they were still low. Steptoe and Edwards had reported an early success rate of 2% per embryo transfer; several years later this rate had risen to 9% per laparoscopy. Other groups in Australia and the United States report rates up to 20%. (3) Notice, though, two different measures of calculation of success rates: per embryo transfer and per laparoscopy. Such lack of standardization makes accuracy of results difficult. Also, the definition of success is not clear. One can be pregnant chemically in that a rise in hormones can be measured, or one can be pregnant clinically in that the embryo has actually implanted. Neither of these necessarily results in a live birth, Nor is a pregnancy of twelve weeks, which is the criterion for success, a necessary predictor of a live birth.

A recent story in the *New York Times* gave the success rate of various IVF clinics in that metropolitan area, defining success as a live birth. The rates for women under the age of thirty-nine ranged from a low of 9.3%, through about 20% at four clinics, to a high of 34% at one clinic. (4) In general, though, of the 267 clinics that report their data to the Society for Assisted Reproductive Technology, the professional association for individuals involved in IVF, the success rate is 21.2% per IVF cycle. (5)

GENERAL ETHICAL ISSUES

The costs associated with IVF raise several ethical issues. Rebate programs, at first flush, sound like a good idea. But some describe this as "at best an eye-catching marketing gimmick, and at worse a breach of medical ethics." An American Medical Association task force argued: "Such publicized guarantees manipulate and unfairly attract patients." (6) For example, Pacific Fertility Center charges $7,725 for its basic, single IVF cycle, while its rebate plan costs $12,500 and up. The plan looks good if one does not become pregnant on the first try, but there is a much more rigorous screening program for people to enter the rebate program, based on one's age and the nature of fertility problems. The desperation for a child may cause individuals to overlook costs or not to do a careful examination of costs or entrance criteria to various rebate plans. It is true that doctors in such programs may do more to enhance the odds of a pregnancy and that the plans can save a couple some money. But they can also lose money if they do not examine all of the fine print: for example, there is no rebate if there is a pregnancy loss after the twelfth week.

The discussion of success rates of IVF procedures also raises ethical issues. I have already noted the problems associated with the lack of common definitions of success as well as of pregnancy, and the choice of one standard over another can greatly increase one's success rate. And this leads to a second problem: the use of such success rates as the basis for advertising, which leads to an increase in clientele and, in turn, to greater income for clinics. IVF clinics appear to be the "only branch of medicine doing success-rate advertising on this scale." (7) Five clinics have had to change advertising claims because of Federal Trade Commission interventions. While most people know to be at least moderately suspicious of advertising claims, these appeals are being made to a rather large and also desperate and vulnerable audience. While such individuals should not be prevented from attempting to have a child, clinics can be held to a strict disclosure standard for both success rates and the basis of their calculations.

A third ethical problem is related to the so-called older woman seeking IVF. Success rates for women forty and older drop by a half to three-quarters of the average rate; these women therefore need very specific information on success rates. Moreover, an increase in the number of women over forty seeking IVF has given rise to a market in eggs from younger women. Some of these come from younger women who successfully underwent IVF and did not need all the eggs that were harvested. Others come from egg donor programs that pay women several thousand dollars to undergo egg retrieval. Such eggs are now part of the advertising campaign. For example, in the 13 January 1997 issue of the *New Yorker,* the Genetics and IVF Institute in Fairfax, Virginia, advertised the availability of almost 100 fully screened donors. While it is true that men have sold their sperm for decades for this purpose, the procedures for egg retrieval are dramatically different and expose the donor to the possibility of both short- and long-term health risks.

THE ROMAN CATHOLIC ETHICAL PERSPECTIVE: *DONUM VITAE*

In this section, I want to turn to a different, and perhaps unlikely, source for an evaluation of some ethical aspects of AR: the 1987 *Instruction* from the Congregation for the Doctrine of the Faith, *Donum Vitae* (DV). This source is unlikely because it prohibits almost every procedure in the area of AR. While I will eventually argue for the rejection of the core of *DV's* natural law argument, there are perspectives in this document that are helpful in evaluating the cultural context in which AR occurs as well as the culture of the clinics themselves. I will identify *DV's* opposition to AR and then turn to a discussion of its positive contributions.

The core argument is a reverse application of the traditional ethical argument used to prohibit artificial contraception. The argument is a classic natural law perspective which says, in the case of contraception, that to separate artificially the act of intercourse from its inherent biological reproductive teleology is to separate what God intended to be united. To separate the unitive and procreative dimensions is to violate the natural integrity of the total act of intercourse. When applied to assisted reproduction, the identical argument is used, but only in reverse. That is, to attain egg and sperm and to unite them in a petri dish and then to implant the zygote is artificially to break apart the inherent unity of the act of intercourse. Or to use the words of *DV*:

> The Church's teaching on marriage and human procreation affirms the "inseparable connection, willed by God and unable to be broken by man on his own initiative, between the two meanings of the conjugal act: the unitive meaning and the procreative meaning." (8)

Citing *Humanae Vitae,* the Congregation goes on to say that "it is never permitted to separate these different aspects to such a degree as positively to exclude either the procreative intention or the conjugal relation."(9) Finally, the Congregation identifies the key ethical flaw in both artificial contraception and artificial conception:

> Contraception deliberately deprives the conjugal act of its openness to procreation and in this way brings about a voluntary dissociation of the ends of mar-

riage. homologous artificial fertilization, in seeking a procreation which is not
the fruit of a specific act of conjugal union, objectively effects an analogous separation of the goods of marriage. (10)

Essentially the argument of *DV* met the same fate as that of its predecessor
and source, *Humanae Vitae.* The majority of commentators, Catholic and
non-Catholic alike, reject the primacy given to a biological structure over the
personal dimension of the act of married intercourse. This overly biological
reading of natural law fits uneasily with the ethical standard suggested in the
Vatican II document *Gaudium et Spes,* which suggests that the moral norm is
to be "the nature of the human person and his acts." (11) Many would argue
that the key to moral analysis is whether the marriage as a whole is open to
procreation, not whether an individual act is. And even here, the tradition
notes exceptions. Beginning with *Casti Connubi* and continuing through *Humanae Vitae,* valid reasons for avoiding conception (without the use of artificial contraception of course) included the health of the mother and the need
to care for the welfare and education of one's current family. And much earlier Thomas Aquinas noted that reproduction was an obligation that fell on
the species, not on any particular individual.

There is an irony in the moral analysis within *DV*: within the context of a
marriage, two individuals *are* attempting to have a child. That is the object
and intent of everything done within the context of AR. *DV* focuses only on
the physical integrity of the act of sexual intercourse and ignores "the fact that
husband and wife are seeking to become father and mother," (12) which of
course is what the tradition says is a goal of marriage. Why the physical integrity of the act should take moral priority over the intention of the husband
and wife to become mother and father through the use of their own genetic
material is both unexplained and unclear.

While the core argument of *DV* may be misplaced or wrong, the document
does raise other features that can be helpful in thinking about the development and practice of AR. For example, *DV* recognizes that, thanks to scientific and medical progress, we have many more effective therapeutic resources available to us. But the document also notes that we "can acquire new
powers, with unforeseeable consequences, over human life at its very beginning and in its first stages." (13) While *DV* uses this to argue for the prohibition of almost all reproductive technologies, that is not its only application.
Research protocols do include the consideration of consequences, and therapeutic interventions are monitored for problems. But typically the focus is
whether the intervention or procedure solves the problem. This occurs because our culture is results-oriented: we want to solve the problem and we
want to solve it now—or yesterday. Only when unforeseen or unintended
consequences occur does the focus shift. As I have noted, very little research

was done on IVF in humans before various procedures were put into widespread clinical application. Fortunately, the outcomes did not prove to be problematic with respect to the well-being of the children born of these processes and, generally speaking, with respect to the well-being of the women utilizing the procedures. But that may be a matter of luck.

Nor should AR be used as a precedent for rapid clinical application of the next technology to be developed. We have a strong bias in this country to act and to refrain from critiques of people's actions. *DV* notes that we are faced with the "temptation to go beyond the limits of a reasonable dominion over nature." (14) The Congregation is not arguing that we should not intervene in nature or seek therapeutic relief. Rather it speaks to the dangers of overreach and of not thinking carefully before we act. *DV* also notes that values cannot come exclusively from the science or technology itself:

> It would on the one hand be illusory to claim that scientific research and its application are morally neutral; on the other hand one cannot derive criteria for guidance from mere technical efficiency, from research's possible usefulness to some at the expense of other or, worse still, from prevailing ideologies. (15)

Science and scientific research are not neutral activities. They are engaged in to achieve certain ends, and these ends are based on particular values. We need to examine why this particular line of research, why this particular project, why this application. And in answering these questions we may learn that there are competing values—for example, service to the patient versus income stream. Certainly, individuals involved in IVF want to provide their patients with the best service possible. However, infertility is approximately a $350 million a year business. Competition for clients is keen. There is also competition between clinics to recruit successful physicians who must then achieve even higher success to justify their salaries. In this context, primacy is not necessarily given to a patient's best interest. We need to go beyond the science of IVF and the values it bears to provide an appropriate evaluation of the practice.

Additionally, the Congregation argues that "an intervention on the human body affects not only the tissues, the organs and their functions, but also involves the person himself on different levels." (16) Later, it approvingly quotes Pope John Paul II: "Thus, in and through the body, one touches the person himself in his concrete reality." (17) This points to several critical issues in contemporary medicine and particularly in assisted reproduction.

One is the tendency of modern medicine to objectify the body (18), which began with the Cartesian perspective that the body was a machine. The Enlightenment tradition consolidated this perspective by focusing on the person as the essential self with the body as an external element, a machinelike addition. This reintroduced a Platonic dualism into philosophy that had been to a large extent overcome by Christianity's insistence on the unity of the person and the subjectivity of the body. For Christianity, it is only the living unity, a substantial union of body and soul, that is the person.

The important point here is that modern medicine has a philosophical perspective built into it. Ironically, that perspective has helped bring about enormous advances in modern medicine. Surgery, organ transplantation, the many visualization technologies, genetic engineering, and AR all rely, to some degree, on seeing the body as an object, as a composite of interchangeable parts or the sum of its parts. The problem occurs when we forget that this perspective has an embedded ideology that leads us to see ourselves in one dimension only: as object. Of course, one comes to the physician because of a problem and the desire to have it solved. But the problem exists within a person and may also raise a host of personal or psychosomatic issues. The particular problem can be solved technically, but the personal issues may remain.

For example, a man may discover that he has a low sperm count and that is the reason for the infertility. While a single sperm may be implanted in the egg and fertilization accomplished, he may feel inadequate, and such inadequacy may in fact be heightened by the continual presence of the child. Or the various tests and procedures for IVF may become routinized, and less attention paid to the woman who experiences these procedures and whose anxiety may be increasing as she gets deeper into the process. The procedures are not neutral somatic experiences. They are done in the context of biological abnormalities and a cultural context that disapproves of childlessness. If, additionally, they are done in isolation from the person's hopes, fears, and expectations, the person can be harmed even though the treatment was successful.

Particularly with IVF, there is the assumption that to cure the disease, repair the damage, or to circumvent the problem is to heal the person. The various technologies of AR, when successful, resolve childlessness but not infertility. Will the infertility that caused the childlessness still be a problem for the individual thus afflicted, as I noted above in the case of a man with low sperm count? Will the use of donor sperm or donor egg have an effect on the individuals or the couple? Or will the joy of the child remove any such difficulties? The fact that a pregnancy has been achieved does not necessarily resolve the totality of the problems associated with infertility: issues of identity, psychosocial integration, and, perhaps, feelings of inadequacy because of infertility.

An analogy is frequently made between individuals who achieve pregnancy through AR and those who have an ongoing condition such as diabetes, depression, or visual impairment. The symptoms of these chronic conditions may be resolved, but the underlying problem is not. Though insulin corrects the blood sugar and drugs may lift the depression, their very use and presence is a daily reminder of one's problem. A decline in the ability to focus one's eyes for reading is a normal consequence of aging and is easily correctable by a trip to the local drug store; nonetheless, the fact of our new and daily dependency on these glasses is a constant reminder of our aging. While some may take this in stride, for others it may be a major developmental crisis.

Thus the larger issue is the perception of the self and how that is related to the outcome of the treatment. For some, achieving a pregnancy and live birth may be enough. For others, the resulting child is a source of joy, but one's inability to do this without technical assistance may be a constant source of frustration, Infertility, even though resolvable, may be a severe blow to one's self-esteem. My point here is not to argue against the use of AR, but to remind us that we continuously need to think of the totality of the person, not just the biological functioning or the technical elements of a solution. If the main focus is on the techniques, if the biology becomes the center of attention, then IVF becomes much more production than reproduction. If the couple and their needs are kept to the foreground as much as possible, then the couple has a context in which to base and understand all the procedures that they will undergo. A great many of the procedures in which they will participate are very impersonal—and that is the way they must be. But if they can be made part of a larger process, grounded in the couples' relationship and their desire for a family, then some of the depersonalization can be softened and the impersonality of the procedures humanized. Even obtaining sperm, obviously not a high tech procedure in most cases, can be very depersonalizing and difficult if thought of as a procedure and not within a personal context. Even having one's partner present or involved in the process maintains the presence and reality of a relationship. This affirms the procreative dimension much more than being sent to a room to "obtain a sample."

The couple using IVF is essentially doing what another couple is doing without IVF: cooperating in the creation of a new being from their love and their bodies. From a moral perspective, there is no difference between IVF and physical intercourse. The psychological difference, which has moral overtones, is that given the conditions under which IVF occurs there is a danger of depersonalization, of stressing the means over the end. What is critical here is the context in which IVF is done and keeping one's attention on the couple, their relationship, and their desire for a family. While this will not ease all the tension, eliminate the pain, or resolve all the frustrations that come with IVF, the couple will at least have a critical moral center in which to understand what they are doing.

Finally, we need to consider the language of assisted reproduction. This term describes the procedure correctly. But there is a critical nuance between reproduction and procreation. Reproduction is a language of manufacture; it is a language of commodification. Procreation is the language of persons and personal engagement. Our language can shape our thinking, and if we use terms that connote objectification we may begin to think in terms of objectification. Of course, all the acts performed in AR are objectifications of the body or body parts. I am not arguing that such a process renders the acts unethical or invests them with a deep ethical flaw. But there is a tension between the technological procedures and language of IVF and its personal outcome. The former can make us forget the latter as well as serve to restructure our thinking because of the language we use to describe the process. The language and the techniques of IVF can help us forget that to touch the patient is to touch the person.

MINING THE RESOURCES

Let me conclude by reflecting on some broader issues related to Roman Catholicism, social ethics, and issues of public policy. I will not necessarily be arguing for a normative position on AR; Roman Catholicism has such a position, and I disagree with elements of it, as noted above. Rather, I will excavate the fundamental weaknesses of the official sexual ethic of Roman Catholicism and show why its social ethics are a better resource for responding to assisted reproduction. My aim is not to present a comprehensive or substantive position on AR, but to mine Catholic ethics for principles that are critical in this public policy debate.

Natural Law

The premise of *Donum Vitae*, as well as that of *Humanae Vitae*, is natural law traditionally understood. Priority is given to biological processes and procedures in understanding the morality of sexual acts. Such a priority is essentially rejected by a majority of contemporary Catholic theologians and ethicists. In *Humanae Vitae* the moral grounding of the argument against artificial contraception is the inseparable connection between intercourse and conception. So too with *Donum Vitae*. As previously noted, such an interpretation rejects or at least diminishes the moral significance of any intentionality on the part of the couple, e.g., to have a child as a part of their marriage, and posits the sufficiency of the physical integrity of the biological act as determinate for the moral evaluation of their actions. In this perspective the goal of a family — at least a traditional part of the understanding of marriage — is held hostage to biology.

The priority of the physical over the personal is deeply imbedded in the modern ecclesiastical tradition. In his book *Love and Responsibility*, written while John Paul II was still Cardinal Karol Wojtyla, we find an example of this framework for the moral evaluation of human acts. The order of nature has its origin in God, "since it rests directly on the essences (or natures) of existing creatures, from which arise all dependencies, relationships and connections between them." (19) Thus the order of nature grounds morality. Or, as John Paul again states it: "But before and above all else man's conscience, his immediate guide in all his doings, must be in harmony with the law of nature. When it is, man is just towards the Creator." (20)

The clear message here is that moral integrity consists in discovering the metaphysical order embedded in the biological order and then conforming ourselves to both. Thus not only does the natural law perspective as represented here call for caution and a sense of limits but also mandates a genuine non-intervention in the biological order. This overly biological view of natural law in turn shapes the Roman Catholic understanding of marriage. The primary focus is on the physical integrity of sexual relations between the couple, rather than how a couple, might achieve a family within the context of their marriage or how marriage might contribute to the social good.

In spite of the efforts of the current Pope to maintain this tradition, a slight, but significant, shift had already occurred. The Second Vatican Council took major strides forward in the theology of marriage by approving Paul VI's teaching that the procreative and unitive ends of intercourse were co-equal, though morally inseparable. This again spoke to the issue of natural law. The council proposed, for example, this as the norm of human activity: "That in accord with the divine plan and will, it should harmonize with the genuine good of the human race, and allow men as individuals and as members of society to pursue their total vocation and fulfill it." (21) This was further specified by the assertion that by the very fact of being created, "All things are endowed with their own stability, truth, goodness, proper laws, and order." (22) The council walked a fine line here, arguing for the integrity of the created order but not that created things are independent of God or that "man can use them without any reference to the Creator." (23) It vacillated between a less biological and a more personalistic understanding of natural law, suggesting that while physical reality is important, one also needs to look at the good of humanity and one's vocation in that context.

This tension was not resolved, as was shown clearly when *Gaudium et Spes* discussed human reproduction.

Therefore when there is a question of harmonizing conjugal love with the responsible transmission of life, the moral aspect of any procedure does not depend solely on sincere intentions or on an evaluation of motives. It must be determined by objective standards. (24)

But the text goes on to say that these standards must be "based on the nature of the human person and his acts." (25) This part of the criterion, while rooted in the tradition, opened the way to a consideration of the person that incorporates more than the biology of his or her acts. But even this opening could not overcome the biologized understanding of natural law as the continuing standard for marital morality.

Given the tension that remained in the documents of Vatican II and the continued assertion of the definitive (some say infallible) character of *Humanae Vitae,* it is no wonder that the priority of the physical over the personal is almost unconsciously assumed as correct. Such an assumption, however, neglects to account for almost thirty years of continuous critique of this position by leading Catholic theologians and ethicists. These critiques focus on whether to define the object of morality as one's intentions or the physical object. Do impersonal structures take precedent over personal acts? Can the goal of a family, which is a major element in the theology of marriage, be frustrated because of malfunctioning biology? The critique continues to recognize the importance of the biological dimension of the person. What it does differently is to argue that the biological should not be understood as a physiological process that is morally normative, but rather as the person's mode of presence in the world, a dynamic and developing reality, a body-self. Through this incarnational presence we are both present to and bound to the world, society, community, and the dynamic of history.

The continued focus on the biological skews the official teaching on marriage by focusing mainly on the sexual—understood mainly but not exclusively as a biological reality—rather than the personal or social-ethical dimension, Traditionally, however, the goods of marriage are defined in terms of sacramentality, family, and personal fulfillment—a formulation going back to Augustine. The focus on sacramentality looks to the presence of grace, expressed and experienced through the mutual love of the partners and to the indissolubility of a valid marriage.

In the current code of canon law, marriage has been redefined as a covenant, not a contract. Covenant is the biblical term used to describe the love between God and Israel, which was extended to the relations between the people of the nation. This makes it possible to reconceptualize marriage within a more dynamic context, a more interpersonal framework, and to emphasize the graced dimension of all aspects of marriage, including the sexual. Thus while much attention is focused on the indissolubility of marriage as a feature of its sacramentality, there is also a critical opening to develop a much more dynamic theology of marriage based on the covenantal union of persons.

Because the concept of covenant extends to the relation between the members of the community, it also carries with it a social dimension. Marriage can model the virtues needed to keep the community together, it can show the service needed to ensure a harmonious community, it can present a constructive use of sexuality, and so on. The roles of marriage in community become constitutive elements of marriage, not just afterthoughts.

Family remains a key issue for Catholics, as indeed it does for growing numbers of individuals and groups within society. A hallmark of traditional Roman Catholic social teaching about the family was that it was the cornerstone and basis of social life. And so it was in pre-Industrial Revolution Western countries. However, after the Industrial Revolution, socialization as well as the production of goods, services, and foods were transferred outside the family. Thus the family changed from the cornerstone of society to one institution among many.

The response of the Catholic church was to try to hold on to its tradition as long as possible, losing many opportunities to construct a teaching that both respected the tradition and responded to changing times. Thus the tradition called for a living wage, but this was defined in terms of what the father of the family should be paid, assuming that the wife/mother would stay with the children. In something of a gesture to contemporary society, *Humanae Vitae* spoke of responsible parenthood—but only within the context of the traditional meaning of natural law.

The consequences of affirming the tradition in spite of a changing social world were twofold. First, the opportunity to address the positive dimension of the new social reality—as well as to critique its shortcomings—was missed. Calls for social reform, such as the emphasis on the living wage, were essentially strategies to restore the family to its status before the Industrial Revolution. Second, the changing role of women was not constructively addressed. Equality between men and women, even in current papal teaching, is defined metaphysically, not in terms of social roles and social conditions. The teaching that was developed was paternalistic; it sought to maintain the women's role as the heart of the family and to protect them from the dangers of the outside world. Teaching about the family, then, has focused on the ethics of reproduction, rather than on creatively developing a theology of the family in the modern world. Encyclicals on women have been written and theologies of marriage and the family have been developed, but these have been done within the traditional context and with the traditional concepts. The argument aims to restore the past rather than to construct the future.

Humanae Vitae did provide some seeds of renewal by officially recognizing that the unitive end of marriage is co-equal with the procreative end. Nonetheless, co-equality of the unitive and procreative still means *co*-equality, and this puts a burden on Catholic couples who discover they are infertile. These couples are told that a family is the fulfillment of marriage but are given few ways to achieve that. Thus, they may feel abandoned by the church at a time when they need the church most. Certainly adoption is an option, and many couples choose it. But the desire for a child of their own creation testifies to the embodied reality of marriage and to their relation with each other. While pregnancy through IVF may be one step removed from pregnancy through physical intercourse, adoption is yet another step removed. Thus for the infertile Catholic couple, the teaching on the co-equality of the procreative and unitive dimension of intercourse returns in a paradoxical way: given the depth of the unity in their marriage, a couple wishes to affirm the procreative dimension. But they are physically unable to do this and are told by the church that they are also morally unable to have children of their bodies through artificial means. Thus the very positive teaching on the place of children in marriage frustrates this couple because they are not morally able to avail themselves of alternative means to this end.

Finally, the church's emphasis on childbearing, intensified by the pronatalist assumptions of American society, inhibits the couple from considering infertility anything other than a loss. Again, a tie to Catholic social ethics might be useful here in helping to remind the couple, as well as the church, that there are other forms of generativity and fruitfulness within the community. While the pain of the loss from infertility will remain, the opportunity to consider these others forms of generativity through a life of service to others might help transform that pain.

Roman Catholic Social Ethics and Reproductive Issues

Over the past century, Roman Catholicism has amassed a rather comprehensive corpus of social teachings in areas such as wage justice, human dignity, human rights, economic justice, justice in the conduct of war, civil rights, and capital punishment. These teachings have had a major impact on American society in a way that the sexual ethic has not: recall the substantive discussions and indeed reactions of the federal government both to *The Challenge of Peace* and *Economic Justice for All*. To some extent, these teachings are built upon the edifice of natural law, particularly in the earlier encyclicals of Leo XIII and Pius XI. But human dignity and rights, based in the nature of the person rather than in biological nature, have played an increasingly critical role, particularly since John XXIII's *Pacem in Terris*. This trend continued, and in Vatican II the document *Gaudium et Spes* identified the person and his or her acts as a legitimate source of morality.

The first and most critical difference between Catholicism's social and sexual ethic is that the sexual ethic, based on the inviolability of biological structure, *admits of no exceptions*. Thus, contraception is always wrong; IVF is always wrong. Social ethics are open to exceptions or compromise because they are based on obligations inherent in the relations of persons and institutions. Killing is wrong, *except* when in self-defense or when ordered by the state as in war or capital punishment. A living wage is mandatory *but* must be calculated with respect to a variety of social and economic circumstances. One way to explain this is to argue that in the field of social ethics, things are more complicated than with sexual ethics. The economic situation of a country is a complex phenomenon; foreign policy involves a host of difficult interactions. To consider these dimensions is not moral relativism, but an acknowledgement that complex situations require complex analysis.

But I would also argue that with regard to sexual ethics, things are not as simple as the tradition would suggest. For example, the decision of whether or not to have a child is a complex one. One or both prospective parents may have a history of genetic disease in their family. The woman may have a medical condition that could compromise her own health during pregnancy. The couple may have debts from their education that they wish to deal with. Or a couple may identify social service as a priority for their marriage. Recognizing that consequences and circumstances have a role in sexual ethics (unfortunately a forgotten part of the Catholic tradition) would go a long way in helping individuals think through in a responsible manner critical decisions they need to make. It would also have the merit of keeping such individuals in contact with the church and its teachings. While there will surely be actions that Catholicism will always prohibit, this approach would provide a more open mode of analysis and a more nuanced argument in that it appeals to a broader normative framework. It would remain faithful to the best instincts of the tradition but would also appreciate the moral dimensions of the dynamic social situation in which we find ourselves.

Roman Catholic social ethics can also make an enormous contribution to the question of health care in this country. Services for various reproductive technologies are but a subset of a much larger question of what services are covered by insurance and the even larger question of who is insured. Currently most people are insured through private payments, employment, or government programs such as Medicare or Medicaid. But there are a large number of individuals who do not fit into these frameworks or who have inadequate coverage. A strong argument for universal coverage can be made from Roman Catholic sources: it is a basic matter of justice to citizens; it is in the best interests of the country as a whole; it is a long-term investment in a healthier population; it is an expression of care for the marginalized. Roman Catholic social ethics can argue strongly that the current system is unjust because so many are uninsured or underinsured, because benefits are distributed in favor of the wealthy or those fortunate enough to have employment, and because prevention is not adequately addressed.

If coverage is a justice question for Catholic social ethics, so too is financing such coverage. Roman Catholic social ethics could make a strong argument for federal funding of such programs, and for a variety of other funding sources. One could argue, as did Pius XI, that the government should provide insurance only until individuals are able to do so for themselves. It could also be argued that insurance is no longer what it was at the time of Pius XI and now should be provided by the state. Wherever one wishes to enter the coverage and funding debate, there are many ethical issues that Roman Catholicism could constructively address.

The more engaging question, given some sort of universal care, is what to include in the basic benefits package. Few would have trouble with a basic package oriented to prevention, with provisions for routine physicals, vaccinations, prenatal care, well-baby care, dietary advice, etc. Such interventions are relatively inexpensive and have long-term benefits. The problem comes when we move beyond these interventions to others, such as expensive diagnostic and screening technologies, organ transplants, kidney dialysis, and assisted reproduction. Procedures like these are in fact provided for by many insurance programs obtained through employment.

How ought reproductive technologies to fare within a system of universal coverage? This question is made difficult because of several unarticulated assumptions on health care held by most Americans: the funding barrel has no bottom; since I have insurance, I'm entitled to everything; quality health care means as much as possible for as long as possible. Catholic social ethics would seriously challenge all of these assumptions. And such a challenge will not be warmly received, as we saw during the disastrous debate over health care in 1993.

Roman Catholic ethics could argue, on the basis of justice and the common good, that access to AR should not be part of a basic package of universal health coverage. First, the shift from the traditional understanding of natural law to a more historically grounded understanding of the person would argue that biological procreation need not have a place of privilege in a marriage. Also, if marriage is no longer a contract that gives partners access to each other's bodies but a covenantal relationship, procreation becomes one among many goods of marriage, not necessarily the defining good. Marriage as a covenant has a more dynamic relation to society; in this context, we could recall the traditional teaching that reproduction is a species obligation, not an individual one. Thus, from a contemporary theology of natural law and of marriage, one can reasonably argue that reproduction is not essential to the integrity of a marriage. And if so, justice claims to including access to assisted reproduction in a basic health care package are weakened.

A second relevant principle is the traditional Catholic concept of the common good. Here one would focus on individual rights in relation to the good of society as well as to the good of the individual. At its best, the concept of the common good is a way to mediate what society and the individual owe each other. One of the strong implications is that, while everyone should be able to participate in social life and to achieve their potential, everyone is not entitled to everything. The concept of the common good would prioritize prevention over cure or, in the case of assisted reproduction, over compensation for a problematic biological condition. It could, in justice, also restrict access to expensive, low success, high risk, nonvalidated therapies. Artificial reproduction is certainly expensive and has a relatively low success rate. Having a family historically has been important for individuals and has been strongly encouraged by the Catholic church along with other religious organizations. Nonetheless, rethinking health insurance will force us to ask how central to individual fulfillment and desire, and how critical to the common good, is having a child of one's own body and partner. Is the provision of basic benefits to all not more important than ensuring that a small group have their reproductive desires fulfilled?

One solution, of course, would be to devise an insurance system so that individuals can, after receiving a basic package, buy other features such as coverage for artificial reproduction. Such a combination of private and public plans would certainly give the wealthy a major advantage. But if it were not totally inaccessible to the less wealthy, it would not be inherently unjust. From the perspective of Catholic social ethics, the key issue would be to ensure that the poor had access to services covered by the basic package. The question of access to other health care options, however, would continue to be welcomed in the context of much larger questions of economic justice within the society.

As I have shown, Roman Catholicism can engage in a very critical public policy debate over AR without making any reference to its sexual ethic, which prohibits AR as unnatural. The more critical Catholic arguments would focus on the relative importance of biological childbearing, funding for research into artificial reproduction, access to reproductive clinics, the place of artificial reproduction in relation to other health care services, and the status and role of children within our society. Catholicism has a vast treasury of social teachings that can be brought to bear on these and other questions, if it lets go of the traditional sexual ethic and develops a moral theology in dialogue with the past, but appreciative of contemporary issues and perspectives. (26)

NOTES

1. *New York Times*, 18 October 1996, sec. B21.

2. Ibid.

3. Clifford Grobstein, Michael Flower, and John Mendeloff, "External Human Fertilization: An Evaluation of Policy," *Science* 222 (14 October 1983): 127.

4. Trip Gabriel, "High-Tech Pregnancies Test Hope's Limit," *New York Times*, 7 January 1995, sec. A10.

5. Ibid., sec. A11

6. Ann Wozencraft, "It's a Baby, or It's Your Money Back," *New York Times*, 25 August, 1996, 3:1.

7. Gabriel, "High-Tech Pregnancies," sec. A11.

8. *Donum Vitae*, II, B.4. The citation can also be found in Thomas A. Shannon and Lisa S. Cahill, *Religion and Artificial Reproduction* (New York: Crossroad, 1988), 161.

9. Ibid.

10. Ibid.

11. *Gaudium et Spes*, para. 51. The document can be found in David O'Brien and Thomas A. Shannon, *Catholic Social Thought: The Documentary History* (New York: Orbis Books, 1992), 200.

12. I am indebted to James Keenan, S.J., for this insight. See his "Moral Horizons in Health Care: Reproductive Technologies and Catholic Identity," in *Infertility: A Crossroad of Faith, Medicine and Technology,* ed. K. Wm. Wides (Netherlands: Kluwer Academic Publishers), 53–71, but especially see 61–62.

13. *Donum Vitae,* Introduction, 1. Also Shannon and Cahill, *Religion and Artificial Reproduction,* 1431.

14. Ibid. Also Shannon and Calill, *Religion and Artificial Reproduction,* 141.

15. Ibid., 2. Also Shannon and Cahill, *Religion and Artificial Reproduction,* 143.

16. Ibid., 3. Also Shannon and Cahill, *Religion and Artificial Reproduction,* 144.

17. Ibid.

18. For an excellent overview of this perspective, see James F. Keenan, S.J., "Christian Perspectives on the Human Body," *Theological Studies* 55 (1994): 330–46. His work illuminated several of my perspectives on this topic.

19. Karol Wojtyla, *Love and Responsibility,* trans. H. T. Willetts (New York: Farrar, Straus, and Giroux, 1981), 246.

20. Ibid., 247. Italics in the original.

21. *Gaudium et Spes,* 209.

22. Ibid.

23. Ibid.

24. Ibid., 229.

25. Ibid.

26. 1 want to thank in a very particular way Kathleen Sands for twice reading this manuscript with a very critical and constructive eye. Her comments have been helpful not only with respect to the organization of the overall argument, but also in terms of pushing the thrust of the argument forward. I am extremely grateful for her editorial and collegial assistance.

4

Sex Selection: Not Obviously Wrong

Bonnie Steinbock

Let me start with the obvious. Sexism and sexual discrimination are bad things. Both sexes have equal human worth, both are entitled to equal treatment and opportunity.

For some people, once we acknowledge these principles, the discussion about sex selection is over. Sex selection is sexism, or it contributes to sexism. As such, it should be morally condemned and discouraged. Some think it should be illegal.

I think this analysis is far too simplistic. Whether sex selection is sexism depends first on what sexism is. Some feminists believe that "gender roles" are all socially imposed and that the rejection of sexism means seeing men and women as basically alike in their abilities, psychology, and characteristics. On this view, anything that treats males and females differently, such as dressing them differently or giving them different names, is sexist. But not all feminists agree. Some think the eradication of sexism does not entail the "no-difference" thesis. Some even think that women are not only different from men, they're better than men, and the world would be a better place if more people displayed feminine virtues of caring, compassion, and patience.

Another element in the discussion of the morality of sex selection is how it is accomplished, whether by preconception means such as sperm sorting, by embryo discard after preimplantation genetic diagnosis (PGD), or by abortion. The motives or reasons individuals have for wanting to determine the sex of their child, and the ways in which these might affect their ability to be good parents, are also relevant. Equally important are the social consequences of permitting sex selection, since choices that may be morally acceptable on the individual level might have harmful social consequences. The social consequences—difficult in any case to ascertain—are likely to differ in different societies. Given the complexity of the issue, a hasty conclusion is unwarranted. Moreover, sex selection is one of those issues, like abortion or pornography, where a "thin" moral analysis, in terms of permissibility or impermissibility, seems very inadequate. (1) A thicker moral discussion of sex selection would include what kinds of attitudes toward gender are desirable, what we should look for in the experience of parenting, and ultimately, what kind of society we should strive to create and what kind of people we want to be.

METHODS OF SEX SELECTION

Abortion

Suppose a couple decides to have a child and the woman becomes pregnant. In a routine sonogram in her seventh month, she discovers, to her surprise, that the fetus is a boy. She is bitterly disappointed. She has always wanted a girl and, perhaps because of this, assumed she was having a girl. She requests a termination so she can "try again" for a girl.

Most people, even those who are strongly pro-choice and want women to have the right to make their own decisions regarding their pregnancies, would find this morally objectionable. Indeed, I think that most people would be horrified. This is partly because most people take a developmental view about the moral status of the fetus. The closer it gets to being born, the stronger are its claims, and the more serious the reasons must be to justify abortion. Most people also differentiate between terminating an unintended and a wanted pregnancy. A woman who becomes pregnant because she wants a child is expected to act "like a mother" to her fetus and her future child. (2) To abort a healthy fetus toward the end of a wanted pregnancy simply because it's the "wrong sex" indicates both callous attitudes toward human life generally and a startling lack of maternal feeling. (3)

These objections to abortion for sex selection do not, of course, apply to preconception methods. The trouble with most preconception methods, which range from folk remedies, such as putting a knife under the pillow to get a boy, to quasi-scientific instructions regarding the timing of intercourse, is that none of them work. Until recently, that is.

Sperm Sorting

A relatively new preconception technology, flow cytometry, trademarked as Microsort, has been successfully used in cattle for more than a decade. The use of flow cytometry in humans started as a way to help couples at risk for X-linked genetic disorders, like hemophilia and Duchenne's muscular dystrophy, which are most prevalent in boys. If such couples could be assured of having a girl, they could be spared the painful decision of whether to terminate a second-trimester pregnancy. The first Microsort baby was a girl born in 1995 to a woman who had lost two brothers and two sons to X-linked hydrocephalus, a fatal swelling of the brain that occurs only in boys. As time went on, however, and word of the technology spread, it attracted the interest of couples who simply preferred children of a certain sex. The Genetics and I.V.F. Institute, where Microsort is performed, had to decide whether to make its experimental technology available to those who wanted to use it for nonmedical reasons. The policy it developed for its clinical trials was that a couple must already have at least one child to be eligible for the program and that they may select a child only of the "nondominant" sex in their family. (4) In other words, Microsort could be used for "family balancing."

In May 2001, the Ethics Committee of the American Society for Reproductive Medicine (ASRM) issued a report that looked carefully at the pros and cons of preconception methods of gender selection and concluded:

> If flow cytometry or other methods of preconception gender selection are found to be safe and effective, physicians should be free to offer [them] in clinical settings to couples who are seeking gender variety in their offspring if the couples 1) are fully informed of the risks of failure, 2) affirm that they will fully accept children of the opposite sex if the preconception gender selection fails, 3) are counseled about having unrealistic expectations about the behavior of children of the preferred gender, and 4) are offered the opportunity to participate in research to track and access the safety, efficacy and demographics of preconception gender selection. Practitioners offering assisted reproductive services are under no legal or ethical obligation to provide nonmedically indicated preconception methods of gender selection. (5)

Preimplantation Genetic Diagnosis

Preimplantation genetic diagnosis (PGD) was developed for couples at risk of having a child with certain genetic diseases. Using IVF, embryos are created and tested for genetic disease. Affected embryos are discarded, and only unaffected embryos are replaced in the woman's uterus to start a pregnancy. PGD has all the disadvantages of IVF: it is expensive, technologically daunting, and imposes significant burdens on the woman. For these reasons, it has only limited use even in the diagnosis of serious genetic disease, (6) much less as a method of sex selection.

It has one great advantage over sperm sorting, however: it really works.

Flow cytometry is still experimental, and probably will never be as accurate as PGD for determining the sex of offspring. With this in mind, Norbert Gleicher, a fertility specialist, asked ASRM if, in light of its position on using sperm sorting for family balance, it would not also be permissible to use PGD. In fact, Gleicher suggested that it would *not* be ethically permissible to offer patients an inferior method when a superior method was available. (7) His institution's IRB agreed.

John Robertson, acting chair of ASRM's ethics committee, said in a letter to Gleicher that it would be acceptable to use PGD for sex selection under the same conditions as those enumerated for sperm sorting. Robertson's letter sparked considerable media attention and elicited shocked responses from fertility experts. "Sex selection is sex discrimination, and I don't think that is ethical," said James Grifo, the president-elect of the Society for Assisted Reproductive Technology. "It's not ethical to take someone off the street and help them to have a boy or a girl." (8) J. Benjamin Youngner, executive director of ASRM, then issued a statement essentially repudiating Robertson's interpretation of ASRM's position. (9) Youngner said that ASRM's position on sex selection was stated in two reports from its Ethics Committee: the above-mentioned May 2001 report and a 1999 report which concluded that PGD solely for sex selection should be discouraged, due to the risk of unwarranted gender bias, social harm, and the diversion of medical resources from genuine medical need.

Youngner did not explain how to reconcile the two reports. Why is sex selection for family balancing acceptable if done using sperm sorting, but unacceptable if done using PGD? One answer might be that sperm sorting is a preconception method, whereas PGD involves embryo discard. As William Schoolcraft of the Colorado Center for Reproductive Medicine expressed it, "With sperm sorting, you are not throwing away potential babies." (10) Many do not regard very early embryos as morally equivalent to babies, of course, but they may believe that embryos have *some* claim on us, requiring that the reasons for discarding them be serious ones. A preference for one sex over the other might not be serious enough.

What if choosing the sex of one's baby is not the reason for undergoing PGD but a side effect? Suppose a couple uses PGD to prevent the birth of a child with a serious genetic disease. Suppose they produce three healthy embryos and only want to implant two, to avoid having a multiple birth. Two of the embryos are female and one male. If they want a girl, would it be wrong to decide which embryo to discard on the basis of sex? I cannot see that it would be, unless having a preference for one sex rather than the other is intrinsically morally objectionable. Reasons for thinking that this is so might be made on either the individual or the societal level.

ATTITUDES TOWARD GENDER

It might be said that the sex of one's child would matter only to someone who has objectionable sexist attitudes—who thinks that little girls should be sweet and quiet, for example, or little boys tough and brave—and will try to impose those views on the child. It is certainly wrong to impose rigid sexual roles on children, but a desire to do so is not the only reason why one might want a child of a particular sex. The desire for a son (let us say) might be based on the recognition that the experience of parenting a boy is different from that of parenting a girl.

To insist that this is not the case seems breathtakingly simplistic, as if gender played no role either in a person's personality or relationships to others. Gender may be partly cultural (which does not make it less "real"), but it probably is partly biological. This was brought home to me when I was wheeling my infant daughter through a drugstore. She spotted a display of toy footballs and reached out to them. Delighted at her nonsexist choice of toy, I said proudly, "Football, Sarah? You want a football?" But when I gave it to her, she immediately held it against her shoulder, patting it gently and saying "Ahhh." Is it plausible that at nine months she had already been indoctrinated into cultural stereotypes? As most parents can attest, at a very young age, boys and girls are attracted to different toys, even when parents make deliberate efforts to give their daughters trucks and their sons dolls. Even when they play with the same toys, the play is often different. This is part of what makes being the mother of a son different from being the mother of a daughter. As someone who has had the good fortune to be both, I see nothing wrong with wanting to have both experiences.

Here it might be objected that there is nothing wrong with *wanting* a girl or *wishing* to have a boy if you already have a girl. What is unnerving is the *longing* that some people experience, and the steps they are willing to take to ensure that they get the sex they want. Is the sex of one's child so important that one is willing to forgo the pleasures and intimacy of sexual intercourse and opt instead for sperm sorting and artificial insemination? Is it worth the expense? It costs $2,500 for each use of Microsort, and the average pregnancy takes three tries. (11) PGD is even more expensive, and involves much greater physical burdens and risks. Even if it is okay to care about the sex of one's child, should one care that much?

These are moral questions. They relate to our ideas about reproduction and sex, what it means to be a parent, what kinds of parent one should strive to be, and what role, if any, gender should have on the parent-child relationship. The importance of these issues is not in doubt. The question is whether these values are primarily personal and individual, or instead merit public discussion and resolution. Many important moral questions are left to individuals: for example, whether to send ones children to private school or to remain within the public schools. Such a decision will affect not only one's own child, but taken with the decisions of others, could eventually have an impact on the entire community. Consider the decision whether to let one's child watch television, how much, and which shows. This too is not a purely "self-regarding" decision.

To what extent should such decisions be left to individuals, and to what extent should they be "communal" decisions? Should health care professionals discuss such matters with parents, or even try to influence their decisions? Should professional societies formulate guidelines and policies in these areas? And if professional societies should discourage using PGD for sex selection, should they be equally concerned about its use for disability, as some disability advocates have argued? (12) In answering this question, we have to think not only about the merits of the arguments against selection for sex and selection for disability, but also about the boundaries of individual liberty and the nature of the relationship between the health care professional and the patient. My point is that the seemingly simple question, "Should people be allowed to determine the sex of their children?" is actually very complex.

I have tried to show that the desire for family balance is not intrinsically sexist or morally objectionable. Nevertheless, as Robert Wachbroit and David Wasserman point out, "individual reproductive decisions may, in the aggregate, have harmful social consequences. . . ."(13) If harmful social consequences were likely to result, they might well overcome considerations based on individual autonomy. If the consequences were likely enough and bad enough, they might justify discouraging or even prohibiting sex selection by any method.

SOCIAL IMPLICATIONS OF SEX SELECTION

Critics of sex selection maintain that it will be used to oppress women. This is not because most people in the United States want to use sex selection to get boys. The opposite may be true. According to a 1999 story in the *New York Times Magazine,* "[o]f the first 111 Microsort attempts, 83 were for females and 28 were for males."(14) This imbalance is partly because Microsort was introduced as a way to avoid diseases primarily affecting males precisely by selecting for girls, and partly because it is just better at selecting for females and so has attracted couples who want them. In addition, however, a growing number of women want daughters and are willing to use technology to "get the girl." How, it may be asked, can sex selection oppress women if it is used to increase the number of baby girls? The answer, Lori

Knowles has suggested, is that biotechnology cannot be confined to one country. "Although the limited experience of Microsort shows a preference for girls within the United States, it will be used in cultures where women are oppressed, and it will be used to select for male children. That will further institutionalize the discrimination against women."(15)

There is no question that sex selection, usually abortion after an ultrasound, is practiced in countries like India and China to ensure the birth of male offspring. In China the population has been so drastically skewed (through abortion and infanticide) that at one point there were 153 boys to every 100 girls. India's 2001 census shows that "the ratio of girls to boys in the richest states of the north and west has fallen sharply over the past decade, a phenomenon that most experts attribute to the rising use of ultrasound tests to determine the sex of a fetus and the abortion of females." (17)

Some argue that such imbalances naturally right themselves, as the dearth of marriage partners for young men makes females more valuable. Others think that something must be done to correct the gender imbalance. The governments of India and China have both banned the administering of prenatal tests solely to determine the sex of a fetus, (18) and the law in India may also apply to preconception sex selection methods. (19)

A ban might reduce the number of abortions for sex selection (though such abortions still get performed), but does it necessarily alleviate the oppression of women? Actually, some women's groups are worried that "curbing sex-determination tests will drive many families back to the centuries-old practice of killing baby girls shortly after birth, or so favoring boys, with scarce supplies of food and other benefits, that girls die young."(20) In a survey concluded in 1995, the National Foundation of India estimated that 300,000 newborn girls die annually from what it called "gender discrimination"—either being killed outright or suffering such neglect that they die of illness or starvation. (21) And this does not take into consideration the harms done to women's health by repeated pregnancies undertaken in the desperate attempt to have a son. Thus well-meaning attempts to fight discrimination against women might actually make them worse off.

But there is a deeper point here as well. Even if there is a correlation in some cultures between sex selection and oppression of women, it does not follow that allowing sex selection causes the oppression of women, or that eliminating sex selection would alleviate the oppression. There may be some third factor that is responsible for both the desire for male children and the oppression of women. Joel Feinberg has made this argument about violent pornography and crimes of violence against women. It seems obvious to some that if we oppose violence against women, we should support laws banning violent pornography. But Feinberg argues, persuasively to my mind, that even if we could establish a significant correlation (as opposed to anecdotal evidence) between men who read violent pornography and men who commit violent crimes against women, that would not prove that the two are causally connected. It is possible that their consumption of violent pornography does not cause them to rape women, but rather that a third factor causes both their preoccupation with pornography and their violence toward women.

This third factor, he suggests, is machismo. Violent porn does not appeal, he says, to normal males, but only to those in the grip of the macho cult. Feinberg goes on to ask, "Would it significantly reduce sexual violence if violent pornography were effectively banned?" He replies that no one can know for sure, "but if the cult of macho is the main source of such violence, as I suspect, then repression of violent pornography, whose function is to pander to the macho values already deeply rooted in society, may have little effect." (22) Similarly, banning sex selection might do little to alleviate the oppression of women, if a sexist ideology is the source both of the oppression of women and the practice of sex selection. In any event, one may be a little skeptical about the wisdom of banning a practice in the United States to keep it from spreading to other countries when it is not even clear that banning the practice in the other countries would benefit women. In an ideal world, women would be valued as much as men, but I personally would prefer to permit people to prevent the births of girls than to see the girls neglected and allowed to die of illness or malnutrition.

We should also consider the possibility that allowing people to determine the sex of their children would have harmful effects right here in the United States. It is unlikely that sex selection here would skew the balance of males and females, since most Americans want a boy and a girl. Nevertheless, a study done by Roberta Steinbacher at Cleveland State University found that of those Americans who would use sex selection, 81 percent of the women and 94 percent of the men would want their firstborn to be a boy. Lori Andrews has commented that this finding is troubling in light of research on birth order, which "consistently finds that first-borns are more aggressive, more achieving, of higher income and education than later-borns. We'll be creating a nation of little sisters." (23) Andrews probably exaggerates here, since the same study found that only 25 percent of Americans would use sex selection. Nevertheless, if sex selection became widely available, it might change the American family, making older sisters to younger brothers somewhat less common than they otherwise would be. Whether this change would be harmful enough to justify constraining choice, however, is hard to say.

Some would argue that it is not choosing the sex of one's child per se that is worrisome, but rather the idea that parents can choose their off-spring's attributes. Children are not cars, it is often said, and they should not be ordered "to spec." Wachbroit and Wasserman make this connection. "Sex selection is only the tip of the iceberg," they write, "deceptively unthreatening because of the broad consensus in this country against the practice and the negligible demand for it. . . . [T]he real threat comes from the identification of an increasing number of genetic markers associated with conditions that are not life-threatening, but impairing or socially undesirable, such as hyperactivity, homosexuality, and obesity. The availability of prenatal tests for those conditions threatens to make pregnancy ever more tentative and to further stigmatize those with the conditions tested for." (24)

But Wachbroit and Wasserman are not offering an argument against sex selection. Sperm sorting would not make pregnancy more tentative, and it is unlikely that allowing parents to have daughters would stigmatize those born with a Y chromosome. Rather, they are offering a reminder that we are entering an age in which prospective parents may have a greater ability than ever to shape their offspring's characteristics. There is the potential for a great deal of good with this new ability, but also a great deal of harm. As individuals and members of society, we need to think about what values our choices reflect, and what consequences they are likely to have. Sex selection should not elicit a "knee-jerk" reaction; it should initiate a nuanced discussion of the various complex issues involved.

NOTES

1. M. Little, "The Morality of Abortion," in *A Companion to Applied Ethics,* ed. C. Wellman (Cambridge: Blackwell Publishing Company, forthcoming).

2. For a discussion of maternal obligations to the not-yet-born child, see my *Life Before Birth: The Moral and Legal Status of Embryos and Fetuses* (New York: Oxford University Press, 1992), ch. 3.

3. Some disability advocates think that selective abortion for disability is not very different from abortion for sex selection. See A. Asch, "Real Moral Dilemmas," *Christianity and Crisis* 46, no. 10: 237–40. Reprinted as "Can Aborting 'Imperfect' Children Be Immoral?" in *Ethical Issues in Modern Medicine,* ed. J.D. Arras and B. Steinbock, 5th ed. (Mayfield Publishing Company, 1999).

4. L. Belken, "Getting the Girl," *New York Times Magazine,* 25 July 1999.

5. Ethics Committee of the American Society for Reproductive Medicine, "Preconception Gender Selection for Nonmedical Reasons," *Fertility and Sterility* 75, no. 5 (2001): 861–64, at 863–64.

6. See J.R. Botkin, "Ethical Issues and Practical Problems in Preimplantation Genetic Diagnosis," *Journal of Law, Medicine & Ethics* 26 (1998): 17–28.

7. G. Kolata, "Fertility Ethics Authority Approves Sex Selection," *New York Times,* 28 September 2001.

8. Kolata, "Fertility Ethics Authority."

9. J.B. Youngner, "ASRM Position on Gender Selection," http://www
.asrm.org/Med/Press/genderselection.html, accessed 1 October 2001.

10. Kolata, "Fertility Ethics Authority."

11. Belkin, "Getting the Girl," 28.

12. A. Asch, "Prenatal Diagnosis and Selective Abortion: A Challenge to Practice
and Policy," *American Journal of Public Health* 89, no. 11 (1999): 1649–57.

13. R. Wachboit and D. Wasserman, "Patient Autonomy and Value-Neutrality in
Nondirective Genetic Counseling," *Stanford Law & Policy Review* 6, no. 2 (1995):
103–11, at 110.

14. Belkin, "Getting the Girl," 29.

15. Belkin, "Getting the Girl," 38.

16. Belkin, "Getting the Girl," 28.

17. C.W. Dugger, "A Claim to Help Choose Baby's Sex Sets Off Furor in India,"
New York Times, 23 November 2001.

18. J.F. Burns, "India Fights Abortion of Female Fetuses," *New York Times,* 27
August 1994; J.F. Burns, "New Chinese Law Prohibits Sex-Screening of Fetuses,"
New York Times, 15 November 1994.

19. Dugger, "A Claim to Help Choose Baby's Sex," *New York Times,* 23 November 2001.

20. Burns, "India Fights Abortion," and Burns, "New Chinese Law."

21. Burns, "India Fights Abortion," and Burns, "New Chinese Law."

22. J. Feinberg, *Offense to Others* (New York: Oxford University Press, 1985),
153.

23. Belkin, "Getting the Girl," 38.

24. Wachbroit and Wasserman, "Patient Autonomy and Value-Neutrality," *Stanford Law & Policy Review* 6, no. 2 (1995): 110.

5

Human Immunodeficiency Virus and Infertility Treatment

Ethics Committee of the American Society for Reproductive Medicine

Human immunodeficiency virus (HIV) has infected people of all ages. The fact that the largest group affected (86%), are persons of active reproductive age (15–44 years) underscores the risk of viral transmission to sexual partners and offspring. Because women make up approximately 20% of cases and because HIV has become more prevalent among heterosexual couples than in the past, some infected persons will probably ask their health care providers for advice about and assistance with having children who are free of the virus.

In 1994, the Ethics Committee of the American Society for Reproductive Medicine set forth guidelines concerning patients with HIV who may request or need reproductive assistance. (1) The Committee expressed concern about potential transmission of the virus to an uninfected partner or to the couple's offspring. It also addressed potential problems for the child related to the shortened life span of one or both infected parents. On the basis of these concerns, the Committee recommended that testing for the presence of the virus be offered to all couples requesting reproductive assistance. The Committee also recommended that institutions establish their own written policies on infertility treatment for people infected with HIV. It suggested that physicians counsel couples about the consequences of using potentially infected sperm and discuss the options of donor sperm, adoption, or not having children.

When these guidelines were published in 1994, HIV infection was considered a serious contraindication to establishment of a healthy pregnancy. Since then, understanding and treatment of HIV-infected persons and laboratory techniques for the preparation of virus-free sperm for reproductive assistance have changed substantially. (2–5) With more effective treatment regimens, the death rate has decreased dramatically among persons who become infected.

Several methods of limiting the risk for HIV transmission to partner and

67

offspring have also been developed. For example, zidovudine has reduced the vertical transmission of infection from 16%–24% to 5%–8% when given to HIV-positive pregnant women during the second and third trimesters and to their newborns for 6 weeks. (4, 6–9)

A meta-analysis of studies conducted in North America and Europe concluded that elective (planned) cesarean section added to antiviral treatment would decrease the vertical transmission rate to 2% compared with 7.6% in children of treated women who deliver vaginally. Subsequent studies have found that cesarean section is not needed to lower the risk of transmission if viral levels in the pregnant woman are undetectable. (10–12)

Lack of apparent transmission of HIV to partner or child with intrauterine insemination and IVF with ICSI has been reported for discordant (male-positive) couples. Highly active antiretroviral therapy can lessen the viral burden in a person's serum and semen. Testing of sperm by using a polymerase chain reaction assay has improved the ability to determine whether the virus is present in the washed sperm preparation. (4, 5, 13–15)

In light of these changes in the treatment, and reproductive consequences for men and women who are HIV positive, the Ethics Committee re-examined its earlier guidelines. This paper addresses ethical issues concerning 1) infertility treatment when one partner is HIV positive, 2) infertility treatment when both partners are positive, 3) knowingly conceiving a child who may be born with HIV, 4) HIV testing for couples seeking fertility assistance, and 5) potential risks to the caregivers of patients who are HIV positive.

INFERTILITY TREATMENT WHEN ONE PARTNER IS HIV POSITIVE

The presence of HIV may not affect the reproductive potential of a seropositive person unless he or she is ill owing to an opportunistic infection. The HIV transmission rate to an uninfected partner is estimated to be approximately 1 in 500 to 1,000 episodes of unprotected intercourse. (16) The risk of viral transmission increases dramatically if the HIV-positive partner's viral load is high or if the HIV-negative partner has a concomitant genital infection, inflammation, or abrasions.

If a woman is HIV positive and her male partner is HIV negative, transmission of infection to the male partner can be avoided by using homologous insemination with the partner's sperm. The resulting pregnancy may still pose some risk to the HIV-positive woman and her child, because opportunistic infections occurring during pregnancy can be devastating to the woman and fetus. An HIV-positive woman may require certain medications in the early stages of pregnancy that could have adverse effects on a developing fetus. Amniocentesis, a procedure commonly recommended to women older than 35 years of age, carries the risk of viral transmission to the fetus as the needle is passed through the HIV-positive woman's abdominal cavity into the amniotic sac.

If an HIV-positive pregnant woman is not actively treated with antiviral drugs, the risk of HIV transmission to the infant is greater than 20% regardless of the viral load. Administration of zidovudine to pregnant women and newborns during the first 6 weeks of life can substantially reduce the risk of HIV transmission to 5%–8%. Delivery by cesarean section and avoidance of breast-feeding may further reduce the chance of infection to approximately 2%.

If a man is HIV positive and his female partner is HIV negative, the risk of transmitting the virus to the female partner appears to be reduced but not eliminated by using condoms during sexual activity, except during ovulation. The seroconversion rate was 4.3% in one study of 92 HIV-negative women with HIV-positive partners trying to establish pregnancies through timed intercourse. Two of the women in this study seroconverted during pregnancy, and another two converted in the postpartum period. These four women reported inconsistent condom use by their partners. (14) Even though some HIV-discordant couples have established pregnancies through timed unprotected intercourse without infecting the negative partner or child, this practice is unsafe and is not recommended.

Recent reports have described specific methods for sperm preparation and testing that can substantially reduce the chance of HIV transmission to the female partner and child. In 1998, Semprini et al. (4) reported using a density gradient and swim-up technique to obtain sperm, which were then tested by PCR assays for the presence of HIV. If the final sperm sample tests negative on these assays, it is used for insemination. With this technique, <1% (6 of 623) of the samples tested positive for the virus and were not used. Semprini et al. reported almost 1,600 inseminations of 513 HIV-negative women, from which 228 pregnancies resulted. A follow-up of 97.5% of the women at 3 months and 92% at 1 year revealed that all children older than 3 months of age and all mothers tested were HIV negative. (4)

In 1998, Marina et al. reported similar results in 63 women using a similar method of sperm processing. (14) More sensitive methods to isolate noninfected sperm are currently being tested for clinical use. (3)

The statistics noted above are reassuring, but as previously stated, the seroconversion rate with unprotected intercourse is low. More data are needed to demonstrate the complete efficacy of these sperm preparation techniques. Until then, couples must still be cautioned about the potential risk of HIV transmission to the uninfected partner and to their offspring. Couples seeking the safest methods to prevent transmission of the virus when the male partner is HIV positive should be counseled about using donor sperm, considering adoption, or not having children.

When male-positive discordant couples want to have their own genetically related children, they should be informed of available risk-reduction techniques and encouraged to seek assistance at institutions that can provide the most effective methods of sperm preparation as well as the rigorous testing and treatment necessary to minimize the chance of HIV transmission to partner and offspring. To determine the true efficacy of the chosen method of treatment, these centers should use strict study protocols with proper informed consent and thorough follow-up of patients, partners, and offspring.

INFERTILITY TREATMENT WHEN BOTH PARTNERS ARE HIV POSITIVE

As with any couple presenting for evaluation and treatment, both persons may have normal fertility potential or one or both may have impaired fertility. If an HIV-positive couple asks for medical advice regarding pregnancy, they must be informed about the risks to the pregnant woman and the risk that a child could become infected. If the viral load can be suppressed to undetectable levels in both partners, the couple may have a child who is free of HIV. Aggressive drug therapy with protease inhibitors and other antiretroviral therapy can extend life and improve health in HIV-positive persons; however, it is unknown whether they will ultimately have a normal or near-normal life expectancy. The child may lose one or both parents to AIDS before he or she reaches adulthood.

ETHICAL ISSUES RAISED BY KNOWINGLY RISKING THE BIRTH OF A CHILD WITH HIV

The risk of HIV transmission to offspring can be greatly reduced but not eliminated. This risk raises ethical issues concerning the scope of freedom to reproduce, what can be considered harm sufficient to justify restricting that freedom, and the responsibilities of health care professionals faced with a request to provide services to HIV-infected patients.

Does a couple's desire to have genetic offspring justify the risk of transmitting a serious disease to their child? Although the risk can be reduced in many ways, it cannot be completely avoided. Those who assess the ethics of assisting such patients to have children must address the question of whether offspring born with HIV are harmed despite the preventive steps taken. They must consider that some risk remains that the child will be born with HIV. Until sperm preparation techniques prove completely effective, there may be no way, short of refraining from reproduction altogether, to completely prevent some cases of HIV transmission. In situations in which a child could be born with a serious disease, one can argue that individuals are not acting unethically in proceeding with reproduction if they have taken all reasonable precautions to prevent disease transmission and are prepared to love and support the child, regardless of the child's medical condition. Similarly, one can argue that health care providers are not acting unethically if they have taken all reasonable precautions to limit the risk of transmitting HIV to offspring or to an uninfected partner. It would not, however, be ethically acceptable for a physician, clinic, or institution to proceed with reproductive assistance if they lacked the clinical and laboratory resources needed to effectively care for HIV-positive couples who wish to have a child. In such instances, the medical care provider should refer couples to a center that has these resources.

The ethical issues raised here are similar in some respects to those in couples who know that they are carriers of an autosomal recessive disease, such as Tay-Sachs disease, sickle-cell anemia, or cystic fibrosis. Such couples may choose to take the risk of having an affected child rather than forgo parenthood; adopt; use a gamete donor; or, if a test result is positive, terminate the pregnancy. The risk of transmitting an autosomal recessive genetic disease cannot be reduced below 25%, whereas the risk of HIV transmission can be reduced to a substantially lower number—in some cases, to less than 2%. Health care workers who are willing to provide reproductive assistance to couples whose offspring are irreducibly at risk for a serious genetic disease should find it ethically acceptable to treat HIV-positive individuals or couples who are willing to take reasonable steps to minimize the risks of transmission.

TESTING INFERTILE COUPLES FOR HIV

The Centers for Disease Control and Prevention estimate that approximately 200,000 persons in the United States have undiagnosed HIV. (17) Because most of these persons are of reproductive age, the question arises as to whether practitioners should require HIV testing for all couples seeking medical or surgical reproductive assistance.

Testing for HIV and other sexually communicable diseases is ethically justified for gamete donors to protect the health of the gamete recipients. The Centers for Disease Control and Prevention, the U.S. Food and Drug Administration, American Association of Tissue Banks, and the American Medical Association all strongly recommend HIV testing for every gamete donor. Agencies may mandate testing in the near future. The American Society for Reproductive Medicine practice guidelines recommend that all gamete donors and recipients be tested for HIV and other sexually transmitted diseases and that testing also be offered to the recipients' partners. (18) Testing donors and recipients for potentially transmittable, infectious conditions can be reassuring to all parties involved in assisted reproductive technology and should be strongly encouraged.

It is especially important to test persons who are considered at high risk for HIV infection, such as those who have a history of repeated sexually transmitted diseases, multiple sexual partners without barrier protection, bisexual behavior, or i.v. drug use. Knowing the HIV status of the, at-risk individual or couple before establishment of a pregnancy could enable health care providers to better assist their patients in making safer reproductive choices.

It is ethically appropriate for practitioners to encourage HIV testing for all couples who want to have children, not just those who request infertility treatment. To mandate that people be tested solely because they request medical assistance in having a child would infringe on their personal liberty and introduce a dubious distinction between those who seek treatment for infertility and those who do not.

On the other hand, it may be appropriate to recommend HIV testing as good medical practice since there are means to significantly lessen the chance for HIV transmission to an uninfected partner and to offspring. An analogy is the common practice of recommending that women seeking to become pregnant be tested for rubella immunity because infection during pregnancy could have dire consequences for the fetus. For couples in which the man has unexplained obstructive azoospermia or congenital absence of one or both vas deferens, it is becoming standard practice to recommend testing for mutations of the cystic fibrosis trans-membrane conductor gene to evaluate the risk of having a child with cystic fibrosis. Few people refuse these tests.

Couples should consider HIV testing as part of responsible parenting. Often associated with testing is the presumed stigma of some past sexual or drug-related misbehavior. Clinicians have a responsibility to educate their patients about the possible means by which infections can be acquired and the advantages of knowing the test results before pregnancy is established.

HIV AND THE HEALTH PROFESSIONAL

Health professionals care for patients with serious and potentially contagious diseases, knowing that they themselves could become infected. Knowledge of diseases, combined with careful hygienic practices, has allowed caregivers to lessen that risk. In the late 1990s, the Centers for Disease Control and Prevention identified only 56 persons who had documented occupational transmission of HIV and another 134 people with possible occupational transmission. (19) Most were nurses and laboratory technicians who accidentally inoculated themselves with a patient's blood by a needlestick or were splashed with bloody fluid and had significant mucocutaneous exposure. If standard universal precautions to prevent infectious disease transmission are taken, the risk of virus transmission to medical caregivers is very small and, in itself, is not a sufficient reason to deny reproductive services to HIV-infected individuals and couples. Clinicians have the same obligation to care for those infected with HIV as to care for patients with other chronic diseases. Concern about the public's perception of a clinic or provider that cares for HIV-positive patients is insufficient excuse to deny services.

Clinicians faced with requests for reproductive assistance from persons who are HIV positive should be aware of the 1998 United States Supreme Court decision in *Bragdon vs. Abbott*. (20) The Court ruled that a person with HIV is considered "disabled" and therefore protected under the Americans with Disabilities Act. (21, 22) According to that decision, persons who are HIV positive are entitled to medical services unless a physician can demonstrate "by objective scientific evidence" that treatment would pose "a significant risk" of infection. The Court determined that having HIV was a disability because it interfered with the major life activity" of reproduction due to the risk of transmitting HIV to offspring. Unless health care workers can show that they lack the skill and facilities to treat HIV-positive patients safely or that the patient refused reasonable testing and treatment, they may be legally as well as ethically obligated to provide requested reproductive assistance.

SUMMARY

Human immunodeficiency virus infection is classified as a chronic disease. It is treatable but not yet curable. Significant advances in HIV treatment appear to have delayed the onset of AIDS and its consequences in many, but not all, infected persons. The potential for HIV-positive persons to have uninfected children and not transmit the virus to their partners has been substantially enhanced, but success cannot be guaranteed. Health care providers and HIV-infected persons together share responsibility for the safety of the uninfected partner and potential offspring. When an affected couple requests assistance to have their own genetically related child, they are best advised to seek care at institutions with the facilities that can provide the most effective evaluation, treatment, and follow-up. Alternatively, they may be advised to look to other options and consider donor sperm, adoption, or not having children.

NOTES

1. Special considerations regarding human immunodeficiency virus and assisted reproductive technologies. *Fertil Steril* 1994;62(Suppl 1):85S.

2. Anderson DJ. Assisted reproduction for couples infected with the human immunodeficiency virus type 1. *Fertil Steril* 1999;72:592–4,

3. Politch JA, Xu C, Tucker L, Anderson DJ. Separation of HI-1 from the motile sperm fraction: comparison of gradient/swim-up and double tube technique. [abstract]. In: abstracts of the Scientific Oral and Poster Sessions of the 57th Annual Meeting of the American Society for Reproductive Medicine. Orlando, FL, Oct. 20–25, 2001:S–49.

4. Semprini AE, Levi-Setti P, Ravizza M, Pardi G. Assisted conception to reduce the risk of male-to-female sexual transfer of HIV in serodiscordant couples: an update. [abstract]. Presented at the 1998 Symposium on AIDS in Women, Sao Paulo, Brazil, September 14–15, 1998.

5. Semprini AE, Levi-Setti P, Ravizza M, Taglioretti A, Sulpizoo P, et al. Insemination of HIV-negative women with processed semen of HIV positive partners. *Lancet* 1992;340:1317–9.

6. Connor EM, Sperling R, Gelber R, Kiselev P, Scott G, O'Sullivan, MJ et al. Reduction of maternal-infant transmission of human immunodeficiency virus type 1 with zidovudine treatment. *N Engl J Med* 1994; 331:1173–80.

7. Graham WJ, Newell ML. Seizing the opportunity: collaborative initiatives to reduce HIV and maternal mortality. *Lancet* 1999;353; 836–9.

8. Lindegreen ML, Byers RH, Thomas P, Caldwell B, Rogers M, Gwinn M, et al. Trend in perinatal transmission of HIV/AIDS in the United States. *JAMA* 1999;282:531–8.

9. Mandelbrot L, Brossard Y, Aubin JT, Bignozzi C, Krivine A, Simon F, et al. Testing for in-utero human immunodeficiency virus infection with fetal blood sampling. *Am J Obstet Gynecol* 1996;175:489–93.

10. The mode of delivery and the risk of vertical transmission of human immunodeficiency virus type 1—a meta-analysis of 15 prospective cohort studies. The International Perinatal HIV Group. *N Engl J Med* 1999;340:977–87.

11. Van Vliet A, van Roosmalen J. Worldwide prevention of vertical human immunodeficiency virus (HIV) transmission. *Obstet Gynecol Surv* 1997;52:301–9.

12. Stringer JS, Rouse DJ, Goldenberg RL. Prophylactic cesarean delivery for the prevention of perinatal human immunodeficiency virus transmission: the case for restraint. *JAMA* 1999;281:1946–9.

13. Marina S, Marina F, Alcolea R, Exposito R, Huguet J, Nadal J, et al. Human immunodeficiency virus type 1—serodiscordant couples can bear healthy children after undergoing intrauterine insemination. *Fertil Steril* 1998;70:35–9.

14. Marina S, Marina F, Alcolea R, Nadal J, Exposito R, Huguet J. Pregnancy following intracytoplasmic sperm injection from an HIV-1-seropositive man. *Hum Reprod* 1998;13:329–47.

15. Peckham C, Newell ML. Preventing vertical transmission of HIV infection [editorial]. *N Engl J Med* 2000;343:1036–7.

16. Mandelbrot L, Heard I, Henrion-Geant E, Henrion R. Natural conception in HIV-negative women with HIV-infected partners. *Lancet* 1997; 349:850–1.

17. Guidelines for national human immunodeficiency virus case surveillance, including monitoring for human immunodeficiency virus infection and acquired immunodeficiency syndrome. *MMWR Morb Mortal Wkly Rep* 1999;48 (RR-13):1–27, 29–31.

18. Guidelines for gamete donation. *Fertil Steril* 1993;59 (Suppl 1):1S–9S.

19. HIV/AIDS Surveillance Report, Centers for Disease Control and Prevention, National Center for HIV, STD and TB Prevention, Divisions of HIV/AIDS Prevention: Surveillance of healthcare workers with HIV/AIDS, June 30, 2000. Available at http://www.cdc.gov/hiv/pubs/facts/hewsurv.htm.

20. *Bragdon v. Abbott* (1998);524 U.S. 624, 118 S. Ct. 2196.

21. Americans with Disabilities Act of 1990. S. 933 One hundred and first Congress of the United States of America at the second session, begun and held at the city of Washington on Tuesday, the twenty-third day of January, 1990.

22. Annas, G. Protecting patients from discrimination—The Americans with Disabilities Act and HIV infection. *N Engl J Med* 1998;339:1255–9.

6

Low and Very Low Birth Weight in Infants Conceived with Use of Assisted Reproductive Technology

Laura A. Schieve, Susan F. Meikle, Cynthia Ferre,
Herbert B. Peterson, Gary Jeng, and Lynne S. Wilcox

Infants who have low birth weight, either because of early delivery or because of fetal growth restriction, are at increased risk for short- and long-term disabilities and death. (1, 2) The use of assisted reproductive technology is an important contributor to the rate of low birth weight in the United States because it is associated with a higher rate of multiple birth, (3, 4) which, in turn, is associated with low birth weight. (5) By 1997, the use of assisted reproductive technology accounted for more than 40 percent of triplets born in the United States. (4) In addition, studies have suggested that there is a higher rate of low birth weight among singleton infants conceived with assisted reproductive technology than among naturally conceived singleton infants (6–8) or among all infants in the general population. (9–13) However, these studies had methodologic limitations. In particular, they did not address the issue of whether infants born as singletons were conceived as part of a multiple gestation that was later reduced either medically or spontaneously to a singleton pregnancy.

In addition, it remains unclear whether the risk of low birth weight among singleton infants conceived with assisted reproductive technology is a direct effect of the procedure involving such technology (14, 15) or reflects some other factor related to the underlying infertility of the couples who conceive using these procedures. (16–18) Studies have been limited by small sample sizes and lack of data regarding such potentially confounding variables as the factors causing infertility and their severity.

We used population-based data from records of procedures performed with assisted reproductive technology in the United States to compare the risk

77

of low birth weight among infants conceived with assisted reproductive technology with that found in the general population. The large sample and detailed data on the procedures and resulting pregnancies provided an opportunity to analyze outcomes according to several important factors, including the number of infants born, the number of fetuses early in the pregnancy, cause of infertility, and factors involved in treatment.

METHODS

Study Population

Clinics and medical practices in the United States are required to report data on every procedure involving assisted reproductive technology to the Centers for Disease Control and Prevention (CDC). (19) Each year, the Society for Assisted Reproductive Technology collects data on such procedures performed in clinics in the United States and provides these data to the CDC. Procedures involving assisted reproductive technology are defined as procedures for the treatment of infertility in which both oocytes and sperm are handled outside the body; these include in vitro fertilization with transcervical embryo transfer, gamete and zygote intrafallopian transfer (in which gametes or zygotes are transferred into the fallopian tube rather than the uterus), frozen embryo transfer, and donor-embryo transfer. Data abstracted from patients' records and submitted to the CDC include each patient's demographic characteristics and medical history, as well as clinical information on the procedures performed and resultant pregnancies and births. In 1996, 300 clinics reported more than 60,000 procedures; in 1997, 335 clinics reported more than 70,000 procedures. Five to 7 percent of clinics that were in operation during these years did not report data, despite the federal requirement; because most of these were known to be small practices, we estimate that the data reported represent more than 95 percent of all procedures performed with the use of assisted reproductive technology.

We included in the present analysis infants conceived through procedures performed in 1996 and 1997 in which the mother was between 20 and 60 years of age. Of 136,972 procedures, 23 percent (31,767) resulted in the delivery of one or more liveborn infants. Because some of these were multiple-birth deliveries, the total number of infants was 45,886. Although a delivery could include both liveborn and stillborn infants, we excluded from our analysis the 182 stillborn infants. A total of 3241 infants with missing data on birth weight were also excluded. Our final sample included 42,463 infants conceived with assisted reproductive technology.

Internal Comparisons

We classified infants according to the number at birth (singleton, twin, triplet, or quadruplet or higher-order birth). Although only liveborn infants were included in this study, the assignment of the number born was based on the total number of liveborn and stillborn infants delivered. Within each birth-number group we examined the risk of low and very low birth weight. Birth weight was recorded as a categorical variable in 500-g strata. We defined low birth weight as 2500 g or less and very low birth weight as less than 1500 g.

We assessed variations in risk according to maternal and treatment-related factors, using stratification and multivariable logistic regression. The factors we evaluated included the number of fetal hearts observed on early ultrasonography (i.e., the number of fetuses in the pregnancy), maternal age, parity, primary cause of infertility, previous procedures involving assisted reproductive technology, and the type of procedure that resulted in the current conception. Procedures were classified according to whether the embryos had been fertilized during the current procedure (i.e., were fresh) or had been previously fertilized and frozen until the current procedure and whether the source of the oocytes was the mother herself (nondonor) or another woman serving as an oocyte or embryo donor. In addition, procedures in which a woman other than the mother served as a gestational carrier or surrogate were classified separately. Thus, the procedure was categorized as involving fresh embryos and nondonor oocytes, frozen embryos and nondonor oocytes, fresh embryos and donor oocytes, frozen embryos and donor oocytes, or a gestational carrier. We considered separately whether intracytoplasmic sperm injection (a procedure in which a single sperm is injected directly into the oocyte) was used in procedures involving fresh embryos and nondonor oocytes and those involving fresh embryos and donor oocytes.

External Comparison

We compared the observed numbers of low-birth-weight and very-low birth-weight infants conceived with assisted reproductive technology with expected numbers. Expected numbers were calculated with the use of the public-use computer file containing the 1997 birth-certificate data for the United States (on 3,389,098 infants born to women who were 20 years of age or older) (20) and were adjusted to match the age and parity distributions for women who conceived with assisted reproductive technology We computed standardized ratios for low birth weight and very low birth weight by dividing the observed numbers by the expected numbers and calculated 95 percent confidence intervals for each estimate. (21)

To rule out the possibility that the reduction of gestations that had initially involved multiple fetuses might explain a higher rate of low birth weight in singletons, we performed secondary analyses that included only those births in which the number of fetal hearts noted on ultrasonography did not exceed the number of infants who were born. (Data were not available to permit the differentiation of spontaneous reductions from medically induced reductions.) To separate the effects of treatment from underlying characteristics of the patients or embryos, we performed several additional analyses in this subsample. In one analysis, we restricted the sample to infants conceived with the use of donor oocytes among couples without a diagnosis of male-factor infertility, since these infants were considered most likely to have been conceived with healthy gametes. In a second analysis, we restricted the sample to infants born to couples with a diagnosis of male-factor infertility, since women in this subgroup were considered unlikely to have uterine or other infertility-related disease. And in a third analysis, we restricted the sample to infants who had been carried by a gestational surrogate, since these surrogates were presumably healthy women.

Analyses were conducted separately for singletons and twins. In addition, we subdivided low-birth-weight infants into term and preterm infants. Preterm delivery was defined as delivery at less than 37 completed weeks of gestation. We calculated gestational age as the interval from the date of oocyte retrieval and fertilization to the date of birth. For procedures performed with the use of frozen embryos and for other procedures for which the date of oocyte retrieval was missing, the gestational age was calculated as the interval from the date of embryo transfer to the date of birth. To make the estimates comparable with those in the general population, we computed the estimated postmenstrual age (the age according to the last menstrual period) as the gestational age in days plus 14. Term low birth weight was defined as a weight of 2500 g or less with delivery at term; preterm low birth weight was defined as a weight of 2500 g or less with preterm delivery.

To assess the contribution of the use of assisted reproductive technology to low birth weight in the United States, we examined 20,369 infants from our study population who were born in 1997; some had been conceived with assisted reproductive technology in 1996 and some in 1997. For singleton infants, twins, and infants from higher-order multiple births, we divided the number of low-birth-weight and very-low-birth-weight infants conceived with assisted reproductive technology by the total number of low-birth-weight and very-low-birth-weight infants born to women 20 years of age or older in the United States in 1997.

This study was approved by the institutional review board of the CDC; in accordance with federal regulations, the requirement to obtain informed consent was waived for this retrospective analysis.

RESULTS

The study population was similar to the total population of women treated with assisted reproductive technology in terms of the characteristics of the women and the infertility treatment they received (table 6.1). However, some factors associated with higher success rates for assisted reproductive technology—an age of less than 35 years, previous deliveries, no previous procedures involving assisted reproductive technology, and the use of fresh embryos (particularly fresh donor embryos)—were slightly more common among the study population.

A total of 43 percent of the infants in the study population were singletons, 43 percent were twins, 12 percent were triplets, and 1 percent were quadruplets or higher-order multiples. The percentage of infants with low birth weight varied from 13.2 percent among singletons to almost 100 percent among quadruplets or higher-order multiples. The percentage of infants with low birth weight varied with maternal characteristics and treatment-related factors (table 6.2). Singletons were more likely to have low birth weight if there had been more than one fetal heart on early ultrasonography, and twins were more likely to have low birth weight if there had been more than two fetal hearts.

The rate of low birth weight was also higher among singletons and twins born to nulliparous women and women who had no previous procedures involving assisted reproductive technology (table 6.2). Low birth weight was less common in infants conceived by couples with male-factor infertility, conceived with intracytoplasmic sperm injection, or carried by a gestational surrogate. Among triplets, 90 percent or more of the infants had low birth weight, regardless of maternal characteristics or treatment-related factors. The percentages of quadruplets and higher-order multiples with low birth weight are not shown in table 6.2 but were nearly 100 percent in all groups. The results for singletons and twins were materially unchanged after multivariable adjustment for the maternal characteristics and treatment factors listed in table 6.2.

The rate of very low birth weight ranged from 2.6 percent for singletons to 66.9 percent for quadruplets or higher-order multiples. The rate of very low birth weight also varied with maternal and treatment-related factors, but to a lesser degree than the rate of low birth weight did (data not shown).

As compared with all singleton infants born in the United States to women 20 years of age or older in 1997, singletons conceived with assisted reproductive technology in 1996 or 1997 were at increased risk for low and very low birth weight (table 6.3). When the analysis was restricted to infants who

Table 6.1   Maternal Characteristics and Characteristics of Assisted Reproductive Technology Used*

Characteristic	Percentage of All Procedures Involving ART (N=136,972)	Percentage of Procedures That Resulted in a Live Birth (N=31,767)	Percentage of Infants Included in Final Sample (N=42,463)
Age of mother			
20–29 yr	10.5	13.1	14.0
30–34 yr	31.2	37.2	38.4
35–39 yr	35.8	34.3	33.4
40–44 yr	19.2	12.3	11.2
≥45 yr	3.3	3.2	3.1
Parity			
0	76.9	75.6	75.3
1	17.0	18.2	18.5
≥2	6.2	6.1	6.2
Primary cause of infertility			
Female factor	69.4	68.0	68.1
Male factor	23.0	24.2	24.1
Idiopathic	7.7	7.8	7.8
Previous procedures involving ART			
0	49.8	55.2	55.8
1	24.7	23.1	22.7
2	12.1	10.8	10.7
≥3	13.4	11.0	10.8
Type of procedure†			
Fresh embryo, nondonor oocyte	76.3	76.9	78.0
Frozen embryo, nondonor oocyte	14.2	9.9	8.9
Fresh embryo, donor oocyte	6.6	10.3	10.5
Frozen embryo, donor oocyte	2.0	1.7	1.6
Gestational carrier	0.9	1.2	1.1
Use of intracytoplasmic sperm injection‡			
No	61.3	62.1	62.9
Yes	38.7	37.9	37.1

*Data on age, parity, primary cause of infertility, and type of procedure were missing for less than 1 percent of infants; data on previous procedures were missing for 3 percent of infants; and data on the use or nonuse of intracytoplasmic sperm injection were missing for 6 percent of infants. The final sample included all live-born infants with data on birth weight. ART denotes assisted reproductive technology.

†Procedures were classified according to whether the embryos had been fertilized during the current procedure (i.e., were fresh) or had been previously fertilized and frozen until the current procedure and whether the source of the oocytes was the mother herself (nondonor) or another woman serving as an oocyte or embryo donor; procedures in which a woman other than the mother served as a gestational carrier were classified separately.

‡Data are for procedures involving fresh embryos and nondonor oocytes and those involving fresh embryos and donor oocytes only.

Table 6.2 Percentage of Infants with Low Birth Weight (≤2500 g) among Singletons, Twins, and Triplets Conceived with Assisted Reproductive Technology in 1996 and 1997*

Variable	Singletons (N=18,408)	Twins (N=18,399)	Triplets (N=5127)
	% with low birth weight		
Total	13.2	55.2	92.4
No. of fetal hearts on early ultrasonography			
1	12.6		
2	17.6	53.2	
3	25.4	61.1	92.4
4	50.0	70.7	94.4
5	—	70.3	—
≥6	—	89.7	—
Age of mother			
20–29 yr	12.4	61.7	92.4
30–34 yr	13.4	55.3	92.7
35–39 yr	13.1	53.6	91.8
40–44 yr	13.5	51.3	91.0
≥45 yr	12.3	53.5	98.1
Parity			
0	13.7	57.3	93.1
1	11.3	48.4	90.0
≥2	12.4	49.8	90.6
Primary cause of infertility			
Female factor	13.6	56.1	92.4
Male factor	12.2	52.7	93.0
Idiopathic	12.5	54.7	90.4
Previous procedures involving ART			
0	14.3	56.6	93.3
1	11.5	54.0	91.5
2	12.7	53.3	93.2
≥3	11.9	51.1	89.6
Type of procedure†			
Fresh embryo, nondonor oocyte	13.6	56.0	92.1
Frozen embryo, nondonor oocyte	10.5	49.5	92.1
Fresh embryo, donor oocyte	14.0	53.6	94.5
Frozen embryo, donor oocyte	11.8	57.1	97.4
Gestational carrier	8.7	50.0	90.0
Use of intracytoplasmic sperm injection‡			
No	14.3	56.8	92.4
Yes	12.7	54.0	93.0

*Data on age, parity, primary cause of infertility, and type of procedure were missing for less than 1 percent of infants; data on previous procedures were missing for 3 percent of infants; and data on the use of intracytoplasmic sperm injection were missing for 6 percent of infants. The percentage of infants with low birth weight is not provided if there were fewer than 20 infants in the category. Global P values were calculated by the chi-square test and were adjusted for correlations between infants within each birth-number group. Global P < 0.05 for all variables except the age of the mother among singletons and all variables among twins. ART denotes assisted reproductive technology.

†Procedures were classified according to whether the embryos had been fertilized during the current procedure (i.e., were fresh) or had been previously fertilized and frozen until the current procedure and whether the source of the oocytes was the mother herself (nondonor) or another woman serving as an oocyte or embryo donor; procedures in which a woman other than the mother served as a gestational carrier were classified separately.

‡Data are for procedures involving fresh embryos and nondonor oocytes and those involving fresh embryos and donor oocytes only.

Table 6.3   Observed and Expected Cases of Low birth Weight and Very Low Birth Weight among Singleton Infants Conceived with Assisted Reproductive Technologies in 1996 and 1997.*

Variable	Total No.	No. of Cases Observed	No. of Cases Expected†	Standardized Risk Ratio (95% CI)
Low birth weight				
All infants	18,398	2423	1339.4	1.8 (1.7–1.9)
Pregnancies with one fetal heart	16,730	2104	1197.1	1.8 (1.7–1.8)
Use of donor oocytes, no diagnosis of male-factor infertility	1,397	190	119.3	1.6 (1.4–1.8)
Diagnosis of male-factor infertility	2,759	329	195.9	1.7 (1.5–1.9)
Use of gestational carrier	180	16	13.3	1.2 (0.6–1.8)
Very low birth weight				
All infants	18,398	480	263.4	1.8 (1.7–2.0)
Pregnancies with one fetal heart	16,730	408	239.2	1.7 (1.5–1.9)
Use of donor oocytes, no diagnosis of male-factor infertility	1,397	49	23.5	2.1 (1.5–2.7)
Diagnosis of male-factor infertility	2,759	78	38.5	2.0 (1.6–2.5)
Use of gestational carrier	180	0	2.6	—

*Ten infants with missing data on parity were not included in these analyses. CI denotes confidence interval.
†The number of expected cases was calculated by applying the rates of low birth weight from the 1997 U.S. birth-certificate data to the population of infants conceived with assisted reproductive technology. The values were adjusted to account for differences in the distributions of age (in the following categories: 20 to 29 years, 30 to 34 years, 35 to 39 years, 40 to 44 years, and ≥45 years) and parity (0, 1, or ≥2) between the two populations.

were carried by a gestational surrogate the risk was no longer significantly increased, but there were relatively few infants in this group.

We stratified low-birth-weight infants according to whether they were born at term or were preterm (table 6.4). Singleton infants conceived with assisted reproductive technology had a risk of term low birth weight that was more than twice that of singleton infants in the general population, and they had a smaller but still significant increase in the risk of preterm low birth weight. The risk of term low birth weight remained elevated in analyses restricted to subgroups of the study population conceived with presumably healthy gametes or carried by a presumably healthy woman. The risk of preterm low birth weight was no longer increased in analyses restricted to study infants who had been carried by presumably healthy women.

Singletons conceived with assisted reproductive technology and delivered at term tended to be born slightly earlier than singletons in the general population (mean gestational age, 39.1 vs. 39.5 weeks). We therefore further adjusted our analyses for the week of gestation at delivery (37 to 41 or more) in addition to maternal age and parity. This adjustment did not substantially change our findings (adjusted term-low-birth-weight ratio, 2.4; 95 percent confidence interval, 2.3 to 2.6).

Among twins conceived with assisted reproductive technology, the risks of both term and preterm low birth weight were similar to those in the general population of twins. The ratio of the rate of low birth weight at term among twins conceived with assisted reproductive technology to the rate among all twins born at term was 1.0 (95 percent confidence interval, 1.0 to 1.1).

The 20,369 infants conceived with assisted reproductive technology and born in 1997 represented 0.6 percent of the 3,389,098 infants born to women 20 years of age or older in the United States in that year. However, we estimate that the use of assisted reproductive technology accounted for 3.5 percent of the infants with low birth weight and 4.3 percent of the infants with very low birth weight born to women in this age group. The excesses were due in large part to the increased number of infants from multiple births who were conceived with assisted reproductive technology. However, the increased rates of low birth weight among singletons conceived with assisted reproductive technology also played a small part (0.6 percent of low-birth-weight singletons were conceived with assisted reproductive technology, as compared with the 0. 2 percent that would have been expected).

DISCUSSION

Singleton infants conceived with assisted reproductive technology were at increased risk for low birth weight at term relative to singletons in the general population of the United States. This risk was not explained by known differences between the two populations in the distribution of maternal age, maternal parity, or gestational age at delivery. In addition, there was an increased risk even in analyses in which the sample was restricted to infants from pregnancies that had not originated as multiple gestations, infants conceived with gametes from apparently fertile persons, and infants from pregnancies carried by women who were unlikely to have an underlying uterine or other infertility-related disease. Thus, this study suggests that the increased risk of low birth weight in singleton infants born at term who were conceived with assisted reproductive technology may be directly related to such treatments for infer-rtility.

Singletons who were conceived with assisted reproductive technology also had a moderately elevated rate of preterm low birth weight. However, increased risks were not observed among all subgroups; in particular, the risk was not increased among infants delivered by a gestational carrier rather than the mother. These subgroup analyses involved greatly reduced samples and must therefore be interpreted cautiously. However, a possible explanation is that the risk of preterm low birth weight associated with assisted reproductive technology may be related to some underlying condition in the women who undergo procedures involving such technology rather than to the procedures themselves.

The mechanisms underlying the association between the use of assisted reproductive technology and low birth weight among infants born at term remain unclear and warrant further research. The use of human menopausal gonadotropin as part of procedures involving assisted reproductive technology has been associated with increases in insulin-like growth factor-binding protein 1; this protein has been linked to intrauterine growth restriction. (22) During pregnancies initiated with assisted reproductive technology, altered levels of other endometrial proteins and increased rates of structural abnormalities of the placenta have also been found. (23,24) These factors may also contribute to growth restriction. A less direct mechanism is also possible. The use of assisted reproductive technology has been linked to such maternal complications as pregnancy-induced hypertension. (25–27)

Studies also suggest that women who have conceived with assisted reproductive technology are more likely to undergo elective cesarean section, resulting in deliveries that occur earlier than those following spontaneous pregnancies. (6,7,25–27) We did not have data on complications of pregnancy or type of delivery, but we did find that singletons conceived with assisted reproductive technology and born at term were delivered slightly earlier than term singletons in the general population. Adjustment for the week of gestation at delivery did not substantially reduce the risk ratio for low birth weight at term. We observed an excess risk of low birth weight among the singletons conceived with assisted reproductive technology who were born at every week of gestation between 37 and 41 weeks.

Twins conceived with assisted reproductive technology and born at term were not at higher risk of low birth weight than twins in the general population. It is possible that the additional risk associated with the use of assisted reproductive technology is negligible in twin pregnancies, which are already at high risk. Twins conceived with the use of medications for ovarian stimulation but without assisted reproductive technology may also be at increased risk for low birth weight and may have accounted for a sizable proportion of twins in the general population. We do not have data on the use of these medications among the mothers of the general birth cohort.

We did not compare the birth weights of triplets and higher-order multiples in our study population with those in the general population. More than 40

Table 6.4　Observed and Expected Cases of Low Birth Weight Among Term and Preterm Singleton Infants Conceived with Assisted Reproductive Technology in 1996 and 1997.*

Variable	Total No.	No. of Cases Observed	No. of Cases Expected†	Standardized Risk Ratio (95% CI)
Term low birth weight				
All infants	18,182	1180	455.2	2.6 (2.4–2.7)
Pregnancies with one fetal heart	16,530	1059	413.1	2.6 (2.4–2.8)
Use of donor oocytes, no diagnosis of male-factor infertility	1,390	80	42.4	1.9 (1.5–2.3)
Diagnosis of male-factor infertility	2,730	190	66.5	2.9 (2.5–3.3)
Use of gestational carrier	180	8	4.7	1.7 (0.5–2.9)
Preterm low birth weight				
All infants	18,182	1206	859.6	1.4 (1.3–1.5)
Pregnancies with one fetal heart	16,530	1011	780.3	1.3 (1.2–1.4)
Use of donor oocytes, no diagnosis of male-factor infertility	1,390	110	75.7	1.5 (1.2–1.7)
Diagnosis of male-factor infertility	2,730	131	126.1	1.0 (0.9–1.2)
Use of gestational carrier	180	8	8.5	0.9 (0.3–1.6)

*Term infants were defined as those born at or after 37 weeks of gestation, and preterm infants were defined as those born at less than 37 weeks of gestation. Ten infants with missing data on parity and 216 infants (1 percent) with missing data required to calculate gestational age were not included in these analyses; of the infants missing gestational-age data, 37 had low birth weight and 179 had normal birth weight. CI denotes confidence interval.

†The number of expected cases was calculated by applying the rates of low birth weight from the 1997 U.S. birth-certificate data to the population of infants conceived with assisted reproductive technology. Values were adjusted to account for differences in the distributions of age (in the following categories: 20 to 29 years, 30 to 34 years, 35 to 39 years, 40 to 44 years, and ≥45 years) and parity (0, 1, or ≥2) between the two populations.

percent of the triplets and higher-order multiples in the general population were conceived with assisted reproductive technology, and the risk of low birth weight was greater than 90 percent among such infants in both groups.

We estimate that more than 3 percent of the low-birth-weight infants and more than 4 percent of the very-low-birth-weight infants born in 1997 were conceived with assisted reproductive technology — six times the proportions that would be expected on the basis of the frequency of these procedures. These higher-than-expected proportions are largely explained by the increased rate of multiple births. Although the use of assisted reproductive technology did not appear to increase the already high risk of low birth weight among infants from multiple gestations, the increased risk of low birth weight among singletons conceived with assisted reproductive technology and delivered at term indicates that infants from both singleton and multiple births must be considered in assessing the effect of assisted reproductive technology on the rate of low birth weight in the United States.

NOTES

We are indebted to the Society for Assisted Reproductive Technology (SART) for the use of its data-reporting system; and to SART, the American Society for Reproductive Medicine, and Resolve, the National Infertility Association, for their support.

1. Guyer B, Hoyert DL, Martin JA, Ventura SJ, MacDorman MF, Strobino DM. Annual summary of vital statistics—1998. *Pediatrics* 1999;104:1229–46.

2. Alberman E. "Low birthweight and prematurity", in: Pless IB, ed. *The epidemiology of childhood disorders*. New York: Oxford University Press, 1994:49–65.

3. Centers for Disease Control and Prevention, American Society for Reproductive Medicine, Society for Assisted Reproductive Technology, RESOLVE. 1998 Assisted reproductive technology success rates: national summary and fertility clinic reports, Atlanta: Centers for Disease Control and Prevention, 2000.

4. Contribution of assisted reproductive technology and ovulation-inducing drugs to triplet and higher-order multiple births—United States, 1980–1997 MMWR *Morb Mortal Wkly Rep* 2000;49:535–8.

5. Martin JA, Park MM. Trends in twin and triplet births: 1980–97 National vital statistics reports. Vol. 47. No. 24. Hyattsville, Md.: National Center for Health Statistics, 1999.

6. Westergaard HB, Johansen AM, Erb K, Andersen AN. Danish National In-Vitro Fertilization Registry 1994 and 1995: a controlled study of births, malformations and cytogenetic findings. *Hum Reprod* 1999;14:1896–902.

7. Dhont M, De Sutter P, Ruyssinck G, Martens G, Bekaert A. Perinatal outcome of pregnancies after assisted reproduction: a case-control study. *Am J Obstet Gynecol* 1999;181:688–95.

8. Verlaenen H, Cammu H, Derde MP, Amy JJ. Singleton pregnancy after in vitro fertilization: expectations and outcome. *Obstet Gynecol* 1995;86:906–10.

9. Bergh T, Ericson A, Hillensjo T, Nygren KG, Wennerholm UB. Deliveries and children born after in-vitro fertilisation in Sweden 1982–95: a retrospective cohort study. *Lancet* 1999;354:1579–85.

10. FIVNAT (French In Vitro National). Pregnancies and births resulting from in vitro fertilization: French National Registry, analysis of data 1986 to 1990. *Fertil Steril* 1995;64:746–56.

11. Gissler M, Silverio MM, Hemminki E. In-vitro fertilization pregnancies and perinatal health in Finland 1991–1993. *Hum Reprod* 1995;10:1856–61.

12. Friedler S, Mashiach S, Laufer N. Births in Israel resulting from in-vitro fertilization/embryo transfer, 1982–1989: National Registry of the Israeli Association for Fertility Research. *Hum Reprod* 1992;7:1159–63.

13. MRC Working Party on Children Conceived by In Vitro Fertilisation. Births in Great Britain resulting from assisted conception, 1978–87. *BMJ* 1990;300:1229–33.

14. Sundstrom I, Ildgruben A, Hogberg U. Treatment-related and treatment-independent deliveries among infertile couples, a long-term follow-up. *Acta Obstet Gynecol Scand* 1997;76:238–43.

15. Olivennes F, Rufat P, Andre B, Pourade A, Quiros MC, Frydman R. The increased risk of complication observed in singleton pregnancies resulting from in-vitro fertilization (IVF) does not seem to be related to the IVF method itself. *Hum Reprod* 1993;8:1297 300.

16. Henriksen TB, Baird DD, Olsen J, Hedegaard M, Secher NJ, Wilcox AJ. Time to pregnancy and preterm delivery. *Obstet Gynecol* 1997;89:594–9.

17. Williams MA, Goldman MB, Mittendorf R, Monson RR. Subfertility and the risk of low birth weight. *Fertil Steril* 1991;56:668–71.

18. McElrath TF, Wise PH. Fertility therapy and the risk of very low birth weight. *Obstet Gynecol* 1997;90:600–5.

19. Fertility Clinic Success Rate and Certification Act of l992 (FCSRCA), Pub. L. No. 102–493 (October 24, 1992).

20. Natality public use tape. Hyattsville, Md.: National Center for Health Statistics, 1997 (data file).

21. Clayton D, Hills M. *Statistical models in epidemiology*. Oxford, England: Oxford University Press, 1993.

22. Johnson MR, Irvine R, Hills F, et al. Superovulation, IGFBP-1 and birth weight. *Eur J Obstet Gynecol Reprod Biol* 1995;59:193–5.

23. Johnson MR, Abbas A, Norman-Taylor JQ, et al. Circulating placental protein 14: in the first trimester of spontaneous and IVF pregnancies. *Hum Reprod* 1993;8:323–6.

24. Jauniaux E, Englert Y, Vanesse M, Hiden M, Wilkin P, Pathologic features of placentas from singleton pregnancies obtained by in vitro fertilization and embryo transfer. *Obstet Gynecol* 1990;76:61–4.

25. Daniel Y, Ochshorn Y, Fait G, Geva E, Bar-Am A, Lessing JB. Analysis of 104 twin pregnancies conceived with assisted reproductive technologies and 193 spontaneously conceived twin pregnancies. *Fertil Steril* 2000;74:683–9.

26. Maman E, Lunenfeld E, Levy A, Vardi H, Potashnik G. Obstetric outcome of singleton pregnancies conceived by in vitro fertilization and ovulation induction compared with those conceived spontaneously *Fertil Steril* 1998;70:240–5.

27. Tanbo. T, Dale PO, Lunde O, Moe N, Abyholm T. Obstetric outcome in singleton pregnancies after assisted reproduction. *Obstet Gynecol* 1995;86:188–92.

7

Pregnancy in the Sixth Decade of Life: Obstetric Outcomes in Women of Advanced Reproductive Age

Richard J. Paulson, Robert Boostanfar, Peyman Saadat, Eliran Mor, David E. Tourgeman, Cristin C. Slater, Mary M. Francis, and John K. Jain

In vitro fertilization (IVF) with donated oocytes has made pregnancy possible for many women whose infertility cannot be treated by any other means. Oocyte donation was initially developed as a therapy for young women with premature ovarian failure, rather than as a means of overcoming the age-related decline in fertility. However, the high success rates observed with oocyte donation among younger recipients were mirrored in women older than 40 years. (1) Several reports confirmed the efficacy of oocyte donation in the older group, (2–5) and subsequently it was demonstrated that pregnancies could be achieved in women older than 50 years. (6, 7) Oocyte donation gradually became an important tool in the armamentarium of the fertility specialist. During 1998, the last year for which published data are available, 4783 cycles of oocyte donation were reported to the American Society for Reproductive Medicine/Society for Assisted Reproductive Technology Registry. (8)

One of the principal concerns regarding the application of this therapy to women of advanced reproductive age is the incidence of obstetric complications that may arise as a result of the advanced age of these new mothers. The increased incidence of underlying medical disease, decreased cardiovascular reserve, and diminished ability to adapt to physical stress that may accompany aging could combine to increase perinatal and maternal morbidity or even mortality. Retrospective population-based studies have suggested an increased risk of poor pregnancy outcome with advanced maternal age. (9) However, such reports are necessarily confounded by inconsistencies in prenatal surveillance, preexisting medical conditions, and access to appropriate health care. In contrast, when patients of advanced maternal age were followed and delivered their infants in a modern tertiary care center, no increase in adverse outcome was noted. (10) Furthermore, few published series address obstetric and neonatal outcomes in this group. (11–13) Therefore, the purpose of this investigation was to describe the obstetric outcomes of women older than 50 years whose pregnancy was the result of IVF with donor oocytes.

METHODS

All cases of oocyte donation in which the recipient was older than 50 years conducted at the Assisted Reproductive Technologies Program of the University of Southern California during calendar years 1991–2001 were included. This study was approved by the institutional review board of the Keck School of Medicine of the University of Southern California. Outcomes of cycles were ascertained by clinic and hospital chart review and telephone follow-up, if necessary. Up to 9 of the pregnancies and their outcomes have previously been reported. (12–14)

Patients

A total of 77 postmenopausal women aged 50 to 63 years (mean [SD], 52.8 [2.9] years) underwent IVF with donor oocytes. Patient characteristics are summarized in table 7.1.

Precycle screening included history and physical examination, pelvic examination, and Papanicolaou testing. A normal endometrial cavity was required and its presence confirmed by a hysterosal-pingogram and/or a hydrosonogram. Recipients were also required to provide documentation of a normal mammogram, chest x-ray, electrocardiogram, complete blood cell count, chemistry panel, lipid panel, and thyroid-stimulating hormone level. Cardiovascular reserve was confirmed by a tread-mill stress test. Per California state law, all recipients underwent infectious disease screening. A semen analysis was obtained from male partners.

All recipients completed a biopsy cycle to assess endometrial response to exogenous estrogen and progesterone. The hormone replacement regimen has pre-

Table 7.1   Characteristics of Recipients (N = 77)

Characteristic	Mean (SD)	Range
Age, y	52.8 (2.9)	50–63
Gravidity	1.2 (1.7)	0–6*
Parity	0.8 (1.2)	0–4*

*None of the prior pregnancies was the result of in vitro fertilization or other assisted reproductive technologies.

viously been described (1–3) and consisted of oral estradiol and intramuscular or transvaginal progesterone.

All couples underwent a psychosocial consultation prior to initiation of therapy. The purpose of this screening was to identify potential issues regarding unequal genetic participation in the anticipated offspring, adjustment to parenthood at an advanced age, and disclosure to the child of his or her genetic background.

Exclusion criteria comprised any chronic medical condition including hypertension and clinically significant findings in any of the screening criteria.

Donors

Donors were young women who were either self-designated (relatives or friends), or anonymous and compensated, and each was matched 1:1 to each recipient. The mean (SD) age was 27.5 (2.6) years (range, 22–33 years).

All donors underwent psychological screening prior to stimulation. Medical screening included history and physical examination, pelvic examination, and Papanicolaou testing. Infectious disease screening similar to that of recipients, chemistry panels, complete blood cell counts, and lipid panels were also obtained. Controlled ovarian hyperstimulation was achieved with standard pituitary down-regulation with leuprolide acetate and ovarian stimulation with human menopausal gonadotropins or recombinant follicle-stimulating hormone. Oocytes were retrieved by trans-vaginal ultrasound-guided follicle aspiration. When supernumerary embryos were available, they were cryopreserved for potential future transfer.

Pregnancies were diagnosed by rising β-human chorionic gonadotropin levels 9 days after embryo transfer. Clinical pregnancies were defined by ultrasound evidence of a gestational sac. Data were analyzed by analysis of variance and the Fisher exact test.

RESULTS

During this 11-year period, 89 oocyte retrievals resulted in a total of 121 embryo transfers (89 fresh and 32 frozen). The mean (SD) number of oocytes obtained per donor was 17.5 (8.4), and the mean number of fertilized oocytes was 9.3 (5.3). The mean number of fresh embryos transferred during the study pe-

Table 7.2 Pregnancy Data

	No.	Clinical Pregnancy, No. (%)	Deliveries, No. (%)
Fresh transfers	89	38 (42.7)	31 (34.8)
Frozen transfers	32	17 (53.1)	14 (43.8)
Total	121	55 (45.5)	45 (37.2)

riod was 3.7 (2.2), and the mean number of frozen embryos transferred was 3.6 (1.4). The number of embryos transferred during 1 cycle gradually decreased over time from up to 5 embryos in the 1990s to 2.2 embryos on average in 2001.

Pregnancy Data

There were 55 clinical pregnancies for a clinical pregnancy rate of 45.5% (55/121). Of the 77 women in the series, 42 (54.5%) had live births. Three women carried 2 consecutive pregnancies. A total of 42 donors provided oocytes for the 45 deliveries. In 26 cases (58%), the delivery was the mother's first. The total live-birth rate in this cohort, combining fresh and frozen cycles, was 37.2% (45/121). Pregnancy data are detailed in table 7.2.

Among the 3 women who carried 2 consecutive pregnancies, all 3 were in their 50s during both pregnancies, each used the same donor to achieve both pregnancies, and 1 of the 3 women experienced preeclampsia during both pregnancies.

Neonatal Data

Of the 45 live births, there were 31 singletons, 12 twins, and 2 triplets delivered. The multiple gestation rate was 31.1% (14/45). The mean (SD) Apgar scores at 1 and 5 minutes were 8.2 (0.9) (range, 6–10) and 9.1 (0.5) (range, 8–10), respectively. Table 7.3 summarizes the neonatal outcomes with respect to gestational age and birth weight at delivery. The mean gestational ages and birth weights of the multiple gestations were significantly less than those of singletons.

Patient Outcomes

Of all live births, 78% (35/45; 95% confidence interval [CI], 63%–89%) were delivered by cesarean. Of singletons, 68% (21/31; 95% CI, 47%–82%) were delivered by cesarean, 6% (2/31; 95% CI, 1%–21%) by vacuum-assisted vaginal delivery, and 26% (8/31; 95% CI, 12%–42%) by normal spontaneous vaginal delivery. Of multiples, 100% (14/14; 95% CI, 75%–100%) were delivered by cesarean (P<.02) compared with singletons. The cesarean delivery rate was not related to age or prior parity within this cohort.

Table 7.3   Neonatal Outcomes

Outcome	No. of Patients	Gestational Age, Mean (SD) [Range], wk	Birth Weight Mean (SD) [Range], g
Singletons	31	38.4 (2.1) [30.6–41.6]	3039 (703) [1108–4233]
Twins	12	35.8 (2.8) [30.0–40.0]*	2254 (581) [1222–3070]*
Triplets	2	32.2 [31.3–33.0]*	1913 [1165–2500]*

*P<.001 compared with singletons.

Perinatal data were ascertained in 40 of the deliveries. The incidence of mild preeclampsia in this cohort was 25% (10/40; 95% CI, 11%–47%); the incidence of severe preeclampsia was 10% (4/40; 95% CI, 3%–23%). There were no episodes of eclampsia. Among women younger than 55 years, preeclampsia was noted in 26% (8/30; 95% CI, 14%–46%) compared with 60% (6/10; 95% CI, 26%–86%) of those aged 55 years or older. The incidence of preeclampsia was similar among women experiencing their first delivery (34.8% [8/23]; 95% CI, 21%–47%) compared with that of women who were multiparous (35.2% 6/17; 95% CI, 21%47%).

Gestational diabetes required diet modification in 17.5% (7/40; 95% CI, 7%–33%) of patients, and 2.5% (1/40; 95% CI, 1%–8%) of patients required insulin. As with preeclampsia, gestational diabetes was more common among women aged 55 years or older (40% [4/10]; 95% CI, 10%–67%) compared with those younger than 55 years (13% [4/30]; 95% CI, 6%–32%).

One patient who was carrying a singleton experienced premature rupture of membranes at 29 weeks and was hospitalized for 10 days until delivery; 1 patient required delivery of twins at 30 weeks' gestation for acute onset of severe preeclampsia; 1 patient underwent hysterectomy for a placenta accreta; and 1 patient received a blood transfusion after a cesarean delivery for placenta previa. There were no neonatal or maternal deaths.

COMMENT

We have previously reported that recipient age does not appear to play a substantial role in the efficiency of oocyte donation, suggesting that endometrial receptivity is unaltered by age. (1–3) The menopausal uterus is not only receptive to implantation with adequate steroid replacement, but also appears capable of supporting the gestation throughout the term of pregnancy. However, controversy remains whether children conceived as a result of IVF experience a higher risk of being born earlier or at a lower birth weight. Schieve et al (15) conducted a recent population-based study comparing infants born after IVF with general population-based controls. Despite the gestational age of singletons at delivery being similar between the 2 study groups (39.1 vs 39.5 weeks, respectively), the risk of a low-birth-weight infant in the IVF group was 2.6 times that of the general population. Interestingly, there was no difference in the percentage of low-birth-weight infants born to women aged 20 to 29 years compared with women older than 45 years. In our cohort, the mean gestational age and weight of singletons, twins, and triplets observed appears to be similar to those historically reported in spontaneous pregnancies in younger gravidas. (16–18)

As with other reports of pregnancy outcomes after assisted reproduction, (1–8) we observed high multiple gestation rates. Multiple gestations increase both maternal and neonatal morbidity rates, and it would seem prudent to limit the number of embryos transferred in this group. (19) With higher per-embryo implantation rates observed with blastocyst transfers, (20, 21) it may be reasonable to offer women older than 50 years the option of single blastocyst transfer to diminish the risk of multiple gestations.

Data with respect to obstetric outcome in this age group are extremely limited. Narayan et al (11) reported a notable lack of maternal and neonatal complications in 7 women older than 50 years who had conceived naturally. A prior series from our institution reported obstetric outcomes of 17 viable pregnancies in women older than 50 years using oocyte donation. (12) Perinatal and neonatal profiles were similar to those observed in the current series.

Because of our screening criteria, no patients had glucose intolerance or hypertension prior to conception. Nevertheless, we observed a high incidence of gestational diabetes and pregnancy-associated hypertension in this group. Furthermore, the incidence of both complications appeared to be markedly increased in women older than 55 years compared with those aged 50 to 54 years. While neither difference was statistically significant, the trend toward higher complication rates with advancing age appeared to be strong and should be evaluated in larger series.

According to data from the National Center for Health Statistics in 1998, hypertension associated with pregnancy was identified in 3.7% of 146,320 pregnancies that ended in a live birth. (22) In another investigation, the incidence of pregnancy-associated hypertension was 9.6% in women older than 40 years compared with 2.7% in younger gravidas 20 to 30 years of age. (23) The observed rate of 35% in the current study represents an approximate 10-fold increase compared with younger gravidas and at least a 3-fold increase when compared with women older than 40 years. This exaggerated rate may be partly due to the influence of donated gametes, which are immunologically foreign to the recipient. Salha et al (24) reported that preeclampsia was diagnosed in 18.1% of women who received donated gametes compared with 1.4% in age-matched controls. Preeclampsia is also more common among primigravidas, (16) who represented more than half of our patients (26 of 45 deliveries).

An analogous increase in the rate of gestational diabetes with increasing maternal age was reported by Mestman (25) In that series, the incidence of gestational diabetes was reported to be 3.7% in women younger than 20 years, 7.5% between the ages of 20 and 30 years, and 13.8% in women older than 30 years. In the current series, 17.5% of women had gestational diabetes managed by diet, and 2.5% had their diabetes controlled by insulin. This suggests that the trend toward higher rates of gestational diabetes with age continues after 50 years of age and represents a 2- to 5-fold increase in incidence compared with younger women.

We observed an unusually high operative delivery rate in this series. This may be a consequence of the high-risk nature of these pregnancies. A recent series comparing IVF pregnancies with natural conceptions in young women (26) reported the cesarean delivery rate to be more than doubled in the IVF group; among singletons, cesarean delivery was 1.75 times more likely after IVF than after natural conceptions. The high operative delivery rate may also represent a separate phenomenon; it is possible that the older uterus may be less efficient in effecting normal labor and vaginal delivery. Our experience suggests that even carefully screened, healthy women older than 50 years who opt for oocyte donation should be advised of an increased incidence of operative intervention at the time of delivery.

To our knowledge, this report represents the largest single cohort of women completing pregnancies in their sixth decade of life. Within the constraints imposed by the limited power of this study, pregnancy and successful delivery may be expected in healthy women in their 50s. In spite of a marked increase in gestational diabetes and pregnancy-associated hypertension in this carefully screened population of women, favorable maternal and neonatal outcome may be expected with contemporary obstetric surveillance and management. Women who choose to become mothers in this age group may expect a high rate of cesarean delivery. On the basis of these data, there does not appear to be any definitive medical reason for excluding these women from attempting pregnancy on the basis of age alone.

NOTES

1. Sauer MV, Paulson RJ, Lobo RA. A preliminary report on oocyte donation extending reproductive potential to women over 40. *N Engl J Med*. 1990;323:1157–1 160.

2. Sauer MV, Paulson RJ, Lobo RA. Reversing the natural decline in human fertility: an extended clinical trial of oocyte donation to women of advanced reproductive age. *JAMA*. 1992;268:1275–1279.

3. Paulson RJ, Hatch IE, Lobo RA, Sauer MV, Cumulative conception and live birth rate after oocyte donation: implications regarding endometrial receptivity. *Hum Reprod*. 1997:12;835–839.

4. Pantos K, Meimeti-Damianaki T, Vaxevanoglou T, Kapetanakis E. Oocyte donation in menopausal women aged over 40 years. *Hum Reprod* 1993;8:488–491.

5. Serhal PF, Craft IL. Oocyte donation in 61 patients. *Lancet*. 1989;1:1185–1187.

6. Sauer MV, Paulson RJ, Lobo RA. Pregnancy after age of 50: application of oocyte donation to women after natural menopause. *Lancet*. 1993;341:321–323.

7. Antinori S, Versaci C, Gholami GH, Panci C, Caffa B. Oocyte donation in menopausal women. *Hum Reprod*. 1993;8:1487–1490.

8. Society for Assisted Reproductive Technology and the American Society for Reproductive Medicine. Assisted reproductive technology in the United States: 1998 results generated from the American Society for Reproductive Medicine/Society for Assisted Reproductive Technology Registry. *Fertil Steril*, 2002;77:18–31.

9. Lehman DK, Chism J. Pregnancy outcome in medically complicated and uncomplicated patients aged 40 years or older. *Am J Obstet Gynecol.* 1987;157:738–742.

10. Kirz DS, Dorchester W, Freeman RK. Advanced maternal age: the mature gravida. *Am J Obstet Gynecol.* 1985;152:7–12.

11. Narayan H, Buckett W, McDougall W, Cullimore J. Pregnancy after 50: profile and pregnancy outcome in a series of elderly multigravidae. *Eur J Obstet Gynecol Reprod Biol.* 1992;47:47–51.

12. Sauer MV, Paulson RJ, Lobo RA. Pregnancy in women 50 or more years of age: outcomes of 22 consecutively established pregnancies from oocyte donation. *Fertil Steril.* 1995;64:111–115.

13. Sauer MV, Paulson RJ, Lobo RA. Oocyte donation to women of advanced reproductive age: pregnancy results and obstetrical outcomes in patients 45 years and older, *Hum Reprod.* 1996;11:2540–2543.

14. Paulson RJ, Thornton MH, Francis MM, Salvador HS. Successful pregnancy in a 63–year-old woman. *Fertil Steril.* 1997;67:949–951.

15. Schieve LA, Meikle SF, Ferre C, Peterson HB, Jeng G, Wilcox LS. Low and very low birth weight in infants conceived with use of assisted reproductive technology. *N Engl J Med.* 2002;346:731–737.

16. Cunningham FG, Gant NF, Leveno KJ, Gilstrap LC III, Hauth JC, Wenstrom KD, eds. *Williams Obstetrics* 21st ed. New York, NY: McGraw-Hill; 2001.

17. Spellacy WN, Handler A, Ferre CD. A case-control study of 1253 twin pregnancies from a 1982–1987 perinatal data base. *Obstet Gynecol.* 1990;75:168–171.

18. Newman RB, Hamer C, Miller CM. Outpatient triplet management: a contemporary review. *Am J Obstet Gynecol.* 1989;161:547–555.

19. Paulson RJ, Ory SJ, Giudice LC, Schlaff WD, Santoro NF, Coddington III CC. Multiple pregnancies: what action should be taken? *Fertil Steril.* 2001;75:14–15.

20. Gardner DK, Lane M. Culture and selection of viable blastocysts: a feasible proposition for human IVF? *Hum Reprod Update.* 1997;3:367–382.

21. Behr B, Pool TB, Milki AA, Moore D, Gebhardt J, Dasig D. Preliminary clinical experience with human blastocyst development in vitro without co-culture. *Hum Reprod.* 1999;14:454–457.

22. Ventura SJ, Martin JA, Curtin SC, Mathews TJ, Park MM. Births: final data from 1998. *Natl Vital Stat Rep* 2000;48:1–100.

23. Spellacy WN, Miller SJ. Winegar A. Pregnancy after 40 years of age. *Obstet Gynecol.* 1986;68:452–454.

24. Salha O, Sharma V, Dada T, et al. The influence of donated gametes on the incidence of hypertensive disorders of pregnancy. *Hum Reprod.* 1999;14:2268–2273.

25. Mestman JH. Outcome of diabetes screening in pregnancy and perinatal morbidity in infants of mothers with mild impairment in glucose tolerance. *Diabetes Care.* 1980;3:447–452.

26. Hansen M, Kurinczuk JJ, Bower C, Weiss S. The risk of major birth defects after intracytoplasmic sperm injection and in vitro fertilization. *N. Engl J Med.* 2002;346:725–730.

8

Reproductive Tourism as Moral Pluralism in Motion

G. Pennings

We see stories regularly in the media about strange or extreme applications of the new reproductive technologies. One of the first cases to get large media attention was that of the 59 year old British woman who went to Italy to become pregnant. Since then one case after another has been brought to our attention. The English couple who visited a clinic in Italy to have preimplantation genetic diagnosis for sex selection for non-medical reasons; a 62 year old French woman who went to the United States to be inseminated with her brother's sperm; a British woman who crossed the channel to Belgium to have a child with the sperm of her deceased husband; a couple of British male homosexuals who found a surrogate mother in the United States, and so on. In all these cases, people moved from one country to another to get the treatment they desired. Although most instances of "reproductive tourism" picked up by the media are sensational, these cases present a highly distorted picture of the phenomenon as a whole. Most movements are made for treatments such as oocyte donation and known or anonymous sperm donation. It can be predicted that this type of travelling will steadily increase. There are indications that most patients are prepared to go abroad to get the type of treatment they want. (1) The call for national and international measures to stop these movements becomes, however, ever louder. The United Kingdom health secretary said in reaction to the birth of twins to a 59 year old British woman that "we'll renew our efforts to have discussions with other countries as to the examples we set and they can establish ethical controls over some of the dramatic achievements of modern medicine". (2) The legal scholar Nielsen has also stated that both national and international measures are called for to prevent this kind of shopping. (3)

REPRODUCTIVE TOURISM

"Procreative tourism" was first named by Knoppers and LeBris in 1991 to describe the practice of citizens exercising their personal reproductive choices in less restrictive states. (4) It is the travelling by candidate service recipients from one institution, jurisdiction or country where treatment is not available to another institution, jurisdiction or country where they can obtain the kind of medically assisted reproduction they desire. As such, it is part of the more general "medical tourism".

This type of travelling is not restricted to Europe. The same phenomenon occurs in the United States and Australia. In Australia, for instance, the differences in legislation between the states concerning access to reproductive technology services results in differential access by single and lesbian women. (5) As a consequence, women from Victoria have been travelling to New South Wales to benefit from the less restrictive law in that state. (6) The United States have known this phenomenon for a long time, especially for abortions. There are large differences between the American states regarding access to treatment, type of treatment, procedures etc of medically assisted reproduction. (7)

Traveling to obtain a medical service does not necessarily mean that one has to cross national borders. This misconception follows from the term "tourism". Given the connotations of the term, which are negative when considered within a medical context, it would be better to replace it by "reproductive travelling" but it seems a bit late for that now. Tourism mainly refers to travelling for recreational reasons. Indirectly, this connotation devalues the desire motivating the journey: it implies that the fertility tourist goes abroad to look for something exotic and strange. Basically this is a form of travelling from a place where treatment is not available, because of the prevailing rules, to a place where it is available. These rules are not necessarily laws but may also be the personal moral convictions of the health care provider, institutional policy guidelines, and recommendations by committees. In countries without legislation on assisted reproduction, each doctor and clinic decides autonomously whether to provide a certain type of treatment and whether to offer a service to a certain type of patient. In Belgium, for instance, the policies concerning assisted reproduction differ considerably between secular hospitals and catholic hospitals. Patients who fear, or know, that they will not be accepted in a catholic clinic will request treatment in a fertility centre with another moral worldview even if this means that they have to travel to another city or to another part of the country. This option, obviously, only exists in the absence of a restrictive national regulation.

THE CAUSES OF REPRODUCTIVE TOURISM

Within the European Union, a few countries, such as Belgium and Italy, have no or very little legislation concerning medically assisted reproduction. By looking at the patient streams flowing to these countries, one can chart the legal restrictions in the rest of Europe. I will focus on Belgium since I am more familiar with the situation there. The latest national report, which presents the data of the Belgian register of assisted reproduction for 1999, indicates that 30% of the patients receiving in vitro fertilisation (IVF) treatments come from abroad. (8) Approximately 2700 oocyte pickups are performed in Belgium for foreign patients. The proportion is significantly higher when oocyte donation is considered: 60% of all patients requesting oocyte donation are foreigners. In one large centre for reproductive medicine, more than half of the oocyte recipients come from abroad. (9) About 10% of these women come from France. These French patients come for two main reasons: i) the candidate parents want to increase their chances of success—in Belgium, contrary to the practice in France, fresh oocytes can be used (freezing of embryos reduces the success rate), and/or ii) because they do not accept the compulsory "personalised anonymity" which operates in France. (10) Other streams of patients come from Germany, where neither oocyte donation nor IVF with donor sperm is allowed; from the Netherlands because of a maximum age limit for the recipient and because surgically obtained sperm cannot be used, and from France where lesbian couples and single women are denied access to assisted reproduction and where female recipients must be of "reproductive age".

Generally speaking, the main causes of reproductive tourism can be summarised as follows: a type of treatment is forbidden by law for moral reasons; a treatment is not available because of lack of expertise or equipment (like pre-implantation genetic diagnosis (PGD)); a treatment is not available because it is not considered safe enough (for the moment); certain categories of patients are not eligible for assisted reproduction; the waiting lists are too long in the home country; and the costs to be paid by the patients are too high in their home country.

The last point is worth mentioning because the classical argument against reproductive tourism is the inequality of access. Only people with the necessary financial means can afford to look for treatment abroad. Although largely correct, this argument is selectively used. Most countries do not reimburse all costs for all IVF cycles and a large part of the infertility treatments are performed in profit based private hospitals. As a consequence, almost all countries discriminate against patients on the basis of income, even for those interventions that are accepted in their country. Those who use the justice argument should first eliminate the existing financial discrimination. Moreover, when the lower financial cost is precisely the reason for crossing the border, the justice argument is difficult to maintain. The real costs for medically assisted reproduction are significantly lower in Belgium compared to other countries. (11) Reproductive tourism in these circumstances reduces injustice and allows poor people to obtain treatment. Finally, this is a strange argument if used by those who impose the restrictions. They prevent people from getting treatment at home and then say that the movements are unfair because only the rich can go abroad.

There is another argument hidden beneath the previous one. Some people seem to blame reproductive tourists for using the escape route: they should suffer like all the others who do not have the money to travel.

> This raises the question of whether it is equitable, within the EU, that Member States may impose their regulatory choices only on those who cannot afford to 'choose' another regulatory regime, by buying a service in another Member State, or to put it the other way, whether it is equitable that some people can in effect 'buy their way out' of ethical or moral choices given legislative force in their own Member State. (12)

The first question, however, is whether the state is justified in imposing a moral view on citizens who did not consent to these rules and principles. In addition, is it equitable when one member state denies its citizens access to a reproductive service that is considered perfectly acceptable in another member state?

POSSIBLE SOLUTIONS

The matter of legislation in the field of assisted reproduction raises a number of questions concerning the relationship between law and morality. What is the appropriate legal response of a postmodern society, characterised by different groups holding different moral outlooks, to moral conflicts and dilemmas? Under which circumstances should people abide by laws that express the substantive moral position of the majority? Given the complexity of the law/morality relationship, I will not try to give a general analysis of the issue here. I will instead focus on the possible legal ways to reduce or eliminate reproductive tourism. This perspective seems to presuppose that reproductive tourism is the *problem*. The phenomenon can be seen, however, as a *solution* to restrictive legislation. In the latter interpretation, the legal "solutions" reveal which type of legislation causes reproductive tourism.

Internal Moral Pluralism

If the existing legislation or regulation in a country allows all people to obtain the medical service they desire, there is no need for reproductive tourism. The easiest way to eliminate such tourism is by abolishing all forms of restrictive and coercive legislation. The principle underlying this position is that the legislation in a democracy should take into account the moral view of the different groups in society.

> Legislation, at least in a democratic society, reflects, and is supposed to reflect, a compromise between the diverse preferences and interests of the members of that society. . . . Hence, a legislative acceptable compromise can be attained only if some considerable degree of moral agreement can be achieved during the course of the political debate. (13)

The best balance would be to adopt a "soft" law which is mainly focused on safety issues and good clinical practice and does not impose strict prohibitions or obligations on anyone. (14)

Since our postmodern society is characterised by a multitude of moral and religious views, the law should not reflect the substantive moral position of one group.

> When there is an intellectually irresolvable plurality of moral viewpoints, there will not be a common basis for coercive constraints justified uncontroversially in a particular common concrete view of the good life. . . . Therefore their legal prohibition should always be under moral suspicion in a secular pluralist society. (15)

Respect for the moral autonomy of the citizens implies that if reasonable people disagree one should not impose one alternative by law. The absence of a law, as practice in Belgium shows, means that other institutions, such as the fertility clinics make the rules. These small scale operations exist side by side and serve the patients who share their moral convictions. One clinic will serve lesbian couples and thus present a view which maintains and emphasises the right to procreate while the clinic next door will refuse to treat them on the basis of a different view to do with responsible parenthood. People who request treatments not provided by one institution can look for another clinic nearby.

This solution can also be seen as a form of harmonisation (see below). The number of reproductive movements will strongly diminish by aligning international law in a liberal direction. This can be done by introducing the rule that no member state should penalise or forbid a treatment that is allowed and practised in another member state. (16) One could argue that this treatment is part of, and accepted by, at least one European culture. The result of this strategy would obviously be that all national legislation would be down regulated to the level of the most liberal country. Legislation would then express the lowest common denominator. (17) After analysing the Blood case, McGleenan predicted that the jurisprudence of the European Court of Justice regarding article 59 of the European Community treaty would generate a structural downward pressure so that any regulation would gravitate towards the most permissive laws. According to McGleenan, the freedom of movement to receive services "must lead to the conclusion that there should be a community wide policy on reproductive technology" which should include a minimum policy standard. (18) The evaluation of reproductive tourism clearly depends, however, on the appreciation of moral diversity.

Coerced Conformity

Three types of action can be distinguished: 1) only citizens are eligible for treatment; 2) restriction of the liberty of movement; and 3) control and criminal charges against offenders.

Citizenship or Permanent Residence

The amount of reproductive travel can be reduced by countries requesting citizenship or permanent residence as a condition for treatment. The HFE Act 1990 in the UK stipulates in section 30 (3) (b), concerning surrogacy, that: "the husband or the wife, or both of them, must be domiciled in a part of the United Kingdom or in the Channel Islands or the Isle of Man". The condition of citizenship can be justified if the regulation foresees certain measures which would become impractical, uncontrollable or impossible if people moved back to their home country. This would be the case if access to the treatment were conditional on a regular follow up of the children. If no such measures are imposed, however, it is not clear why citizenship should be a condition. If requests by lesbian couples are accepted, then why should foreign lesbian couples be denied access? It is not up to the visited country to enforce moral rules imposed by a neighbouring country if these differ from its own. A possible exception to the unlimited admission of foreigners is the protection of the internal system by keeping the waiting lists within acceptable limits. This applies to oocyte donation where, because of the shortage of oocyte donors, the waiting time may exceed several years. In that case, a limit on the number of foreign applicants can be established to prevent indirect harm being done to one's own citizens. (19) Since the tolerant society is not responsible for the influx of foreign candidates, its residents should not suffer as a result of this influx.

Restriction of the freedom of movement

The state can try to prevent people from crossing the border to obtain treatment elsewhere. Ireland wanted to bar Irish women from leaving the country to obtain an abortion in Great Britain. In 1992, a 14 year old rape victim was restrained from leaving Ireland for nine months but this injunction was later overturned. Although the ban on abortion was maintained, two amendments to the Irish constitution stated that the freedom to travel between states could not be limited and that the freedom to obtain and make available information relating to services lawfully available in another state could not be restricted. (20) Since the authorities generally do not know who is going where for what, the effective application of this rule would demand a complete closure of the borders except for the very young and the very old.

Articles 59 and 60 of the European Community treaty guarantee the free movement of services, including medical services and thus infertility treatment. This implies that people have the right under community law to go to another country and receive the service they desire.

Control and Criminal Charges

A more drastic violation of people's privacy, autonomy, and bodily integrity was adopted by Germany around 1990. German border guards forced gynaecological examinations upon women re-entering Germany at the Dutch border in search of evidence of extraterritorial abortions. Prosecutors also brought criminal charges against women who obtained abortions in other countries. (21) The European parliament condemned these practices in 1991.

International Harmonisation

The regulation of assisted conception can be categorised as to different approaches: the "private ordering approach" (United Kingdom); the "cautious regulatory system" (Denmark); the "prohibitive licensing system" (Austria), and the "liberal constitutional approach" (Canada). (22) The existence of different legal systems renders international harmonisation particularly difficult. (23) When people talk about harmonisation, they seem to think of agreement on a number of acts and treatments which should be prohibited. This idea also underlies the much criticised European Convention on Human Rights and Biomedicine. (24) After studying the regulations in several countries, Knoppers and LeBris (4) identified a number of issues on which a general consensus exists. There are, however, different definitions of consensus (25) and different levels at which the consensus might occur. A consensus might be reached if the principles are defined very broadly without checking whether people also agree on the implications of the principles in concrete cases. Everyone might agree that "respect for human dignity" and "inviolability of the human person" deserve safeguarding but that does not mean that the same conclusions will be reached when surrogacy and embryo research are discussed. The diversity that characterises the moral perspectives on medically assisted reproduction is downplayed for political reasons. Although the European institutions recognise the principle that matters of (bio)ethics belong to the jurisdiction and competence of the member states, the European Convention on Human Rights and Biomedicine is an indirect attempt to reduce diversity and to standardise legislation around a set of moral rules about which there was never a consensus to start with.

Consensus on a list of prohibitions is pointless as long as there is no global consensus. The globetrotters involved in reproductive cloning demonstrate this. A European list of prohibitions will merely change the destinations. Only a worldwide consensus would eliminate the problem and that is, to put it mildly, highly unlikely. The reaction to reproductive cloning nicely illustrates the purpose of national legislation in a world where location is a trifling fact. Some countries have broken law making world records trying to block reproductive cloning. The prime objective of these laws is not, however, to prevent reproductive cloning from happening since there is no way national legislation could do this. The first goal of the law makers was to keep their own hands clean, by preventing cloning from being performed on their territory.

Interstate Moral Pluralism

In a democracy, political parties attempt to organise society according to their goals, values, and principles. The political programmes include ethical or religious convictions. Political parties try to put their moral stamp on the positions expressed in the societal institutions, among which is the law. However, "democracy is not based on the principle of consensus but on the principle of majority". (26) The conflict between the parties and groups is decided by the majority rule in parliament. If the democratic process functions normally the view on the good life of the majority will prevail at the expense of the minority view. This problem will only disappear when the majority includes everyone and consensus becomes unanimity.

What is ethically right or good is not decided by which norms the majority supports (27, 28) but the ethical rules that apply in social life (what is allowed, obliged or forbidden) are, at least partially, decided by the politicians who vote the laws. Neutrality of the state is impossible here. A nation without any regulation or legislation regarding bioethical issues supports the position that each citizen should decide according to his or her personal moral convictions whether a certain treatment is acceptable. This contradicts the view of those who want to prohibit certain applications of the new reproductive technologies. Allowing as well as prohibiting implies taking sides. It is not an option for policy makers simply to do nothing. (29) This political right should be balanced, however, against other values and principles to prevent the development of a dictatorial state that would fit every single part of our social life into one particular conception of the good life. Among these values we count autonomy, tolerance, and mutual respect. A state which uses excessive coercive power to promote majority values will end up permanently suppressing minority groups. (30) There is a difference between organising social life according to substantive moral principles and using all possible means to force each and every citizen to abide by these rules. Tolerance towards people with different moral positions, who express their disagreement in a peaceful manner, should be a characteristic of a pluralist society.

Imposing a moral opinion on persons who do not share this view creates the risk of conflicts which threaten peace and cooperation in society. (31) Since position taking by the state is unavoidable, two stances to reduce the risk of moral warfare can be distinguished. In the first stance, the majority adjusts its position to incorporate some of the objections of the other groups. This leads to a compromise where, for instance, certain acts are allowed but only under certain conditions or certain acts are prohibited except under specific circumstances. Such a compromise, however, is not always possible and is not necessarily experienced as sufficient by the opponents. The second way to diminish conflicts is when the state demonstrates a degree of tolerance towards the dissenting agents who violate the rules. By allowing reproductive tourism, most states show a degree of tolerance. Three conditions should be present before we can talk of tolerance: the state disapproves of the conduct of the tourist (which it shows by forbidding what the tourist is going to do elsewhere); the state has the power to stop or punish the tourist, and the state chooses to allow the violation. (32) The second condition is fulfilled since most states could impose much stricter measures to enforce their position. The examples given above from Ireland and Germany demonstrate this. But also on other points this type of reticence is demonstrated. The third condition is clearly illustrated by Sweden. Sweden thinks that every child born by means of donor insemination has the right to know the identity of its genetic father. This law caused one of the first European streams of reproductive tourism: Swedish couples going to Denmark where donor anonymity is guaranteed. Even though the Swedish government knows that most parents do not tell the child about the way it was conceived (33) (as a consequence, the child cannot ask for the donor's identity), it has, however, chosen not to introduce a measure that would effectively guarantee the child's right to know. The state could for instance state the name of the donor on the child's birth certificate. By not doing so, it tolerates wrongful behaviour on the part of the parents.

Two levels of tolerance are important for the topic of reproductive tourism: internal tolerance, such as the pragmatic tolerance found in the Netherlands (32) and external tolerance, such as reproductive tourism. Internal tolerance allows the violation of the law within the territory by stating that offenders will not be punished under certain conditions while external tolerance allows citizens to escape from the law by travelling outside the territory without being punished or stopped. While internal tolerance can produce legal insecurity for the citizens, external tolerance gives a clear message about what is permitted in the country. The final result of a policy of external tolerance is that a certain norm is applicable and applied in society as wanted by the majority while simultaneously the members of the minority can still act according to their moral view by going abroad. On deeply felt moral issues concerning life and death (such as reproduction, abortion, euthanasia etc), this policy prevents a frontal clash of opinions which may jeopardise social peace. Obtaining the desired treatment by travelling partially defuses the conflict and prevents the frustration and indignation of the minority group from accumulating. More positively, tolerance towards these movements also shows a healthy degree of relativism. The fact that reasonable people in one's home country and the majority in a neighbouring country opt for a different solution should raise a spark of doubt about the correctness of one's own position. Allowing people to look abroad demonstrates the absolute minimum of respect for their moral autonomy.

Within this context, diversity in legislation (combined with reproductive tourism) is beneficial for all. it could be argued that a pluralistic state should respect all positions but, as I mentioned earlier, this comes down to adopting a liberal perspective that ignores the view of those who think that a certain conduct should be prohibited. Harmonisation of a restrictive legislation would close down the option of travelling and thus increases the risk of a violent conflict within the society.

A DIFFERENT CONCEPTION OF LAW AND REGULATION

The diversity of regulation worldwide and the travelling of people across frontiers raises the question whether "any single jurisdiction can continue to enforce its own rules". (34) I would argue that legislation is still useful as a public statement of the moral conviction of the majority of the people of a jurisdiction. if, however, one hopes to achieve through the law that some interventions are no longer performed or that citizens will no longer use certain medical services, then prohibitions are no longer useful. Given interstate travelling, it is impossible to enforce laws that people do not consider morally justified. Those who do not share the moral standards reflected in the law will either go abroad or find other ways to sidestep the legal restrictions. In general, the ability to enforce laws is strictly linked to the territory. This fact already influences the way law makers presently look at new law proposals. The Swiss federal council (35) argued against a referendum initiative that wanted to prohibit most forms of in vitro fertilisation and the use of donor gametes, that the only consequence of such a law would be the flight of infertile couples to neighbouring countries. Instead of leading to fewer applications for the intended interventions, it would only lead to a relocation of the applications. Moreover, this would take away all possibility of control on the part of the state.

An interesting effect of the existence of alternatives for the citizens (diversity means choice) is that the law makers have to put much more effort into trying to convince the people of the acceptability or unacceptability of a certain action. The existence of different views stimulates reflection and obliges the holders of each position to offer rational arguments to convince those who hold the other position. Information campaigns and large public debates on ethical issues will be indispensable. A good illustration of the limitations of the law to change behaviour in the field of medically assisted reproduction is the Swedish law on donor insemination. After 15 years of a law which makes identifiability of the gamete donors mandatory, only 11% of the parents have told their children and this number does not even take into account the number of couples who went abroad during this period to avoid the law. (33) Apparently the parents are not convinced of the rightness of telling in the context of donor identifiability. In this situation, the introduction of more coercive measures without an accompanying effort to convince people by information and debate would only lead to more reproductive tourism and to more frustration.

CONCLUSION

Reproductive travelling is a pragmatic solution to the problem of how to combine the democratic system which proceeds according to the majority rule, with a degree of individual freedom for the members of the minority. Although the majority has the political right to express their view of the good life in legislation, other values, such as tolerance and mutual respect, urge them to use this right moderately. It is preferable within a pluralistic society, when reasonable people disagree on the acceptability of a certain course of action, to look for a legal compromise that takes into account the positions of different moral communities and to avoid as much as possible radical prohibitions. Even if these recommendations are followed, however, moral conflicts will occur. In those cases, respect for the moral autonomy of the minority demands an attitude of tolerance. This minimally implies that the state refrains from taking active measures (such as restrictions on the freedom of movement of, and criminal charges against, offenders) to prevent citizens from seeking medical care in a state that holds a policy that better accords with their moral insights,

NOTES

Research for this article was made possible by grant G0065,00 from the Fund for Scientific Research, Flanders, Belgium.

1. Dolanska M, Evans D. "Patient perceptions of assisted conception services", in: Evans D, ed. *Creating the child*. London: Martinus Nijhoff Publishers, 1996: 291–301.

2. Morgan D. "Licensing parenthood and regulating reproduction: towards consensus?", in: Mazzoni CM, ed, *A legal framework for bioethics*. London: Kluwer Law International, 1998:107–115: 110.

3. Nielsen L. "From bioethics to biolaw", in: Mazzoni CM, ed. *A legal framework for bioethics*. London: Kluwer Law International, 1998:39–52: 40.

4. Knoppers BM, LeBris S. Recent advances in medically assisted conception: legal, ethical and social issues. *American Journal of Law and Medicine* 1991;17: 329–61.

5. Bennett B. Reproductive technology, public policy and single motherhood. *Sydney Law Review* 2000;22:625–35.

6. Button V. Legal bid to bypass fertility ruling. *The Age* 2000 Aug 28.

7. Kreimer SF. The law of choice and choice of law: abortion, the right to travel, and extraterritorial regulation in American federalism. *New York University Law Review* 1992;67:451–519: 458.

8. College of Physicians Reproductive Medicine and the Belgian Register for Assisted Procreation. *Verslag 1998–1999*. Brussels: College of Physicians Reproductive Medicine and the Belgian Register for Assisted Procreation, 2001.

9. Baetens P, Devroey P, Camus M, et al. Counselling couples and donors for oocyte donation: the decision to use either known or anonymous oocytes. *Human Reproduction* 2000;15:476–84.

10. Raoul-Duval A, Letur-Konirsch H, Frydman R. Les enfants du don d'ovocytes anonyme personnalisé. Aspects psychologiques. *Journal de Gynecologie, Obstetrie et Biologie de Reproduction* 1991;20:317–20.

11. See reference 8: 24.

12. Hervey TK. Buy baby: the European Union and regulation of human reproduction. *Oxford Journal of Legal Studies* 1998;8:207–33.

13. Wellman C. "Moral consensus and the law", in: Bayertz K, ed. *The concept of moral consensus.* London: Kluwer Academic, 1994:109–122.

14. Ferrando G. "Artificial insemination in Italy", in: Evans D, ed. *Creating the child.* London: Martinus Nijhoff Publishers, 1996: 255–66.

15. Engelhardt HT Jr. *Bioethics and secular humanism: the search for a common morality.* London: SCM Press, 1991: 129.

16. Sass H-M. Introduction: European bioethics on a rocky road. *Journal of Medicine and Philosophy* 2001;26:215–24.

17. Nielsen L. "Procreative tourism, genetic testing and the law", in: Lowe N, Douglas G, eds. *Families across frontiers.* London: Kluwer Academic, 1996: 831–48.

18. McGleenan T. "Reproductive technology and the slippery slope argument: a message in Blood", in: Hildt E, Graumann S, eds. *Genetics in human reproduction.* Brookfield USA: Ashgate, 1999: 273–83.

19. Pennings G. Distributive justice in the allocation of donor oocytes. *Journal of Assisted Reproduction and Genetics* 2001;18:58–65.

20. Lawson R. The Irish abortion cases: European limits to national sovereignty? *European Journal of Health Law* 1994;1:167–86:180

21. See reference 7. 458.

22. Lee RG, Morgan D. *Human fertilisation & embryology: regulating the reproductive revolution.* London: Blackstone Press Limited, 2001: 268.

23. Nielsen L. "Legal consensus and divergence in Europe in the area of assisted conception—room for harmonisation?", in: Evans D, ed. *Creating the child.* London: Martinus Nijhoff Publishers, 1996: 305–24.

24. Mori M, Neri D. Perils and deficiencies of the European Convention on Human Rights and Biomedicine. *Journal of Medicine and Philosophy* 2001;26:323–33: 325.

25. Wertz DC, Fletcher JC, eds. *Ethics and human genetics: a cross-cultural perspective.* New York: Springer Verlag, 1989: 12.

26. Bayertz K. "The concept of moral consensus: philosophical reflections", in: Bayertz K, ed. *The concept of moral consensus.* London: Kluwer Academic, 1994: 41–58.

27. See reference 26: 47.

28. Kuhse H. "New reproductive technologies: ethical conflict and the problem of consensus", in: Bayertz K, ed. *The concept of moral consensus.* London: Kluwer Academic, 1994: 75–96.

29. See reference 28: 90.

30. Kymlicka W. Liberal individualism and liberal neutrality. *Ethics* 1989;99: 883–905.

31. Engelhardt HT Jr. *The foundations of bioethics.* Oxford: Oxford University Press, 1986.

32. Gordijn B. Regulating moral dissent in an open society: the Dutch experience with pragmatic tolerance. *Journal of Medicine and Philosophy* 2001;26:225–44.

33. Gottlieb C, Lalos O, Lindblad F. Disclosure of donor insemination to the child: the impact of Swedish legislation on couples' attitudes. *Human Reproduction* 2000; 15:2052–6.

34. Brazier M. Regulating the reproduction business? *Medical Law Review* 1999;7:166–93.

35. Conseil Fédéral Suisse. Avis du conseil fédéral. Initiative "pour une procréation respectant la dignité humaine" 2000. http://www.admin.ch/ch/f/pore/va/20000312/explic/index.html.

9

What Are Families For? Getting to an Ethics of Reproductive Technology

Thomas H. Murray

The standard approach to the ethics of reproductive technologies starts and ends with the parents' procreative liberty. There's much more to think about. We should start with the relationship between parents and children.

Procreative liberty, as the regnant contemporary framework for thinking about the ethics of reproductive technologies, has its defects. It begins with a pair of confusions and disregards a central vital interest; it ignores the values at the heart of family life and relies on a thin and unsatisfying conception of human flourishing.

Intellectual frameworks matter: They direct our attention toward certain moral considerations over others, and they implicitly tell us what, like the cents column on income tax returns, can be ignored. Once the shortcomings of procreative liberty as the dominant framework in ethical discourse on assisted reproduction become obvious, so does the need for a more fulsome and nuanced framework, one that begins with the moral significance of the relationship between parents and children, the values at the heart of that relationship, and the ways in which people flourish, or shrivel—physically, emotionally, and morally.

I want to describe briefly the defects in procreative liberty as a framework for thinking about parents and children. I also want to propose a different starting point—a more challenging and complex one to be sure, that begins with what we value most highly and insists on keeping the broader picture in view, however difficult that may sometimes be. Finally, I want to explore what difference it would make to begin with one rather than the other framework.

AN IMPOVERISHED WORLDVIEW

The confusions in the standard account of procreative liberty are twofold. First, procreative liberty seems confused as to its purpose. Does it mean to be an insightful ethical analysis that illuminates what is morally important about families, parents, and children? Or is it only a quasi-moral, quasi-legal algorithm for considering questions about law and policy in reproductive technologies? Its proponents often write as if procreative liberty was indeed a comprehensive moral account of the ethics of initiating parenthood, and implicitly of parenthood in general. (1)

The second confusion abides in the claim that decisions about what sort of child to have and what means to employ to create a child are merely the flip side of decisions *whether* to have a child—that is, decisions about abortion and contraception. Advocates of procreative liberty fix on the free choices of presumably autonomous adults. But abortion and contraception are means *to not have* a child, at least not at this time, or not under these circumstances. The not-so-flip side is the decision *to have* a child, to create a new person who will have interests, hopes, and concerns of her or his own. It is also a decision to initiate a vital, life-long relationship.

The most egregious defect of procreative liberty is its nearly complete disregard of the interests of children created through reproductive technologies. Advocates of procreative liberty accept one side-constraint: it does not justify creating a child who is worse off than if he or she had never been born at all. I have described this as akin to trying to divide by zero—an arithmetic operation that cannot yield a meaningful answer. All we need agree here is that, as a practical matter, this supposed constraint in practice constrains far too little, if it constrains anything at all.

Imagine a couple who ask that the developing spinal column of their fetus be disrupted, making the child paraplegic. Why would they want to do such a thing? Perhaps they desire the experience of raising a child with a disability, perhaps they believe the demands of caring for such a child will help keep their failing marriage together, perhaps they already have a child with paraplegia, desire another, but do not want their older child to feel less capable than its younger sibling or the child-to-be to feel different from its older sibling. We may be curious about the reasons or motivations behind such a request, but procreative liberty disallows interest in reasons and motivation. It is none of your business, procreative liberty declares.

I want to be clear: I do not believe that proponents of procreative liberty embrace the prospect of prenatal mutilation. My point is rather that the conceptual framework they employ provides no firm support for morally condemning such an action. It permits adults to use virtually any reproductive means for virtually any end; it prohibits or condemns almost nothing. The test of an analytic moral framework cannot be limited to those cases for which it gives the answers one wants; if it provides morally dubious or outrageous answers in other cases, or feeble answers where moral judgments should be clear and ringing, then we have reason to doubt its insightfulness and completeness.

The third defect, procreative liberty's failure to acknowledge values at the heart of family life, is the most sweeping difficulty and at the same time the most difficult to remedy. Control and choice—the values at the heart of procreative liberty—are not entirely out of place in the relationship between parents and children. But they are hardly the entire story, or even the most important themes, and excesses of control and choice can distort and destroy what is most precious in families.

FAMILIES, VALUES, AND HUMAN FLOURISHING

The standard account of procreative liberty is truncated and impoverished. It limits its moral universe to a few values, primarily autonomous adult choice and control. Left out are the values served by parenthood and families, and the role that enduring relationships play in our flourishing as human beings.

Advocates of procreative liberty might argue that the decision about which particular values to pursue is left to the adults making the choice. They can point to the analogy with a woman's right to choose whether to become pregnant or to carry that pregnancy to term.

Here, I think, is where procreative liberty makes a fundamental mistake. Whatever one believes about women's moral rights concerning birth control or abortion, it is undeniable that becoming pregnant and giving birth to a child have an enormous impact on women's lives and on their possibilties for flourishing. Having, raising, and loving a child is a profoundly life-altering experience for both women and men. We must not lose sight of this. At the same time, unpredictable and uncontrolled fertility can restrict women's opportunities for education and work; it consigns some women to deep, enduring poverty.

Procreative liberty's problems began when it appropriated the abstract principle—the right to choose—and ripped it out of the rich context that provided its moral heft: women's prospects for flourishing are diminished when they have no control over their fertility. Procreative liberty then applied that abstracted idea to a very different context—parents, children, and families—with little or no reflection on how these affect our flourishing.

We need a richer ethical framework. We need a framework that acknowledges what should be obvious: decisions about *having* a child are not merely the other side of the moral/legal coin of decisions *not to have* a child. Many people—indeed, probably a robust majority of Americans—support women's access to abortion yet have qualms about the commercialization of reproduction, the growing powers of control over the traits of our children, and reproductive cloning. Our framework must acknowledge the moral significance and interests of the children created through reproductive technologies and do so in a full and robust manner, not as a side-constraint that proves meaningless in practice. And this framework must attend carefully to the values central to the relationship between parents and children, and not be satisfied with the valorization of choice and control in the hands of autonomous adults.

Having and raising children is not the only way to find the enduring, intimate relationships that typify families. But it is the path chosen by many, including those who use reproductive technologies. There are central human values that are either found only in the context of enduring, committed human relationships such as families, or that rely upon such relationships for their realization. Values such as love, loyalty, intimacy, steadfastness, acceptance, and forgiveness are crucial to well-functioning families, which are also the most robust settings in which to raise children to become confident, competent, loving, and emotionally resilient adults.

I do not mean to romanticize families: families can be driven by selfishness, betrayal, and mistrust, or shattered by injustice and oppression. Humans are fallible and all families are imperfect. Yet families are also astonishingly powerful communities of shared memory and experience. Those memories can be scorching and bitter—consider children who were victims of sexual abuse within their family. But they can also be sweet or, perhaps as powerful an emotional glue, a bittersweet mingling of disappointment and loss with love and enduring mutual constancy.

HOW WE GOT HERE

The roots of our current way of framing the ethics of reproduction are old and deep, manifested in the nascent bioethics movement in the latter half of the twentieth century. As bioethics began to gather steam as a field of scholarly inquiry with an accompanying commentary on practical ethical issues, there arose parallel social and political currents concerning women's reproductive capabilities, the emergence of effective and reasonably safe means for controlling those capabilities, and with those new means of control, new possibilities for women's lives. Women could now think about what a good life for them would entail, a good life that had no need to deny a central role to having, raising, and loving children, yet one that also envisioned creative work and other activities outside the household, activities that uncontrolled fertility made difficult or impossible.

The availability of reliable and reasonably safe and convenient contraception has been credited with leading to a sharp change in sexual mores. But that may be looking through the wrong end of the telescope. Contraception, and then in 1973 the legalization of abortion, gave women the means to avoid having a child when for whatever reason they did not want to. What also happened, particularly in the wake of the U.S. Supreme Court decision in *Roe v. Wade,* was that different views of women's nature and flourishing had now been laid out for all to see and had become pivotal in the fierce debates and policy battles over abortion.

Less attention has been paid to differences in the conceptions of men's flourishing, but those differences are every bit as important. As Kristen Luker has written, people's views about abortion were woven deeply into a complex fabric of beliefs, not least about what constituted flourishing for women and for men, and how disparate those two conceptions were from each other. (2) For several years when my children were very young, I cared for them as a single parent, and when Cynthia and I met and married, we cared together for them, including a daughter born from our marriage. The caring I experienced from my own parents—father as well as mother—prepared me well to care for—and enjoy profoundly—my children. A sharp division of capacities between men and women has never struck me as convincing. Women can be more or less competitive; so can men. Men can be better or worse nurturers; the same for women.

Reflections such as these have convinced me that we must take seriously conceptions of human flourishing if we are to have any chance for meaningful moral dialogue or robust and sensible public policy on a variety of issues concerning conceiving, bearing, and raising children. Any wise inquiry into ideas about human flourishing must acknowledge diversity. It must also, I believe, pay great attention to the similarities and the disparities between the conceptions held about flourishing for women and for men.

It would be unforgivably foolish to presume that all people everywhere shared the same notions of human flourishing. The Taliban, for one, made very sharp distinctions in their perceptions of good lives for women and for men, differences that are likely to reflect and be reflected by assumptions about the nature of women and men. As this example suggests, diversity must be given its due—but not more than its due. If you ask your neighbors where they find meaning in their lives, they will tell you in overwhelming numbers that it is in their families. If you talk with someone who has recently had their first child, as my daughter Kate and her husband Matt did with Grace Emilia, our first grandchild, they are likely to tell you—through the haze of exhaustion—that the experience is life-transforming and wondrous.

None of this is peculiar to post-industrial America. In his stunning scholarly tour de force, *The Kindness of Strangers: The Abandonment of Children in Western Europe from Late Antiquity to the Renaissance,* the late historian John Boswell wrote:

> Everywhere in Western culture, from religious literature to secular poetry, parental love is invoked as the ultimate standard of selfless and untiring devotion, central metaphors of theology and ethics presuppose this love as a universal point of reference, and language must devise special terms to characterize persons wanting in this 'natural' affection. (3)

And I can agree with Thomas Jefferson who wrote to his daughter of his hope that his granddaughter "will make us all, and long, happy as the center of our common love." (4)

The awful price that must be paid for this profound attachment, when a child dies, is the enormous, life-long grief that comes in its wake. People say that the death of your child is the worst thing that can happen to a person. Our experience affirms the truth of that.

Of course, there are families in which deep affection never takes hold, or loses out to selfishness or indifference. And there are times and places when grinding poverty and uncontrolled fertility led to the abandonment of many children who could not be cared for. But the fact that all parents are imperfect and some downright awful, and that some families are blighted by poverty or illness or oppression or any of a multitude of factors that can stunt the growth of love and mutual concern, should not blind us to what is morally and emotionally important about families, to the central role families play in many people's flourishing.

We will find better insight about what it means to be human, I believe, by reflecting on the central relationships in our lives and the significance of those relationships for our flourishing, than by focusing exclusively on the liberty of autonomous adults. We must take care to acknowledge and understand differences among conceptions of flourishing, but we should not reflexively set aside the best and most broadly shared understandings of human flourishing simply because no single one commands universal accord. (5)

Those different conceptions lie barely beneath the surface of some of our most bitter public disputes, yet we regularly fail to acknowledge or probe for possible areas of agreement. The obvious example is the debate over abortion, where the disputants prefer to battle over intractable metaphysical questions about the moral status of fetuses and embryos or the limits of state control over women's bodies. These are important questions, to be sure, but they are not the only wedges into the broader disagreements. They are merely the ones that allow partisans on both sides to feel righteous.

It is neither likely nor desirable that only one rich, full-fledged conception of human flourishing prevail in our public policy debate. But I do believe that failing to engage each other about competing conceptions of human flourishing and the values central to family life results in a moral debate in which many of the most important elements remain hidden or scarcely noticed. It likewise results in public policies that are fiercely resisted—as in abortion—or virtually non-existent—regrettably true of reproductive technologies in the United States (a lack that makes us an object of curiosity in other countries). The divide between right-to-life and pro-choice factions in the United States has resulted in an enormous hole in American public policy. Any political leader who takes on the world of infertility treatment, IVF, and the like does so at risk of his or her political life.

WHERE TO START THINKING

In practice, procreative liberty and what we could call a flourishing-centered approach diverge especially in what moral considerations they include. Take, for example, the case of the Nash family. Their daughter, Molly, would die without a life-saving infusion of healthy, immunologically compatible blood stem cells. One possible source: the stem cell-rich umbilical cord blood from a new brother or sister. The Nashes used preimplantation genetic diagnosis for two simultaneous purposes—to avoid having another child with Fanconi anemia, a life-threatening illness, and to choose an embryo that might become, upon birth, a compatible cord blood donor for its older sister. Procreative liberty dictates a two-step analysis: Was this choice an authentic, informed expression of the prospective parents' autonomy? Would the child have been better off never being born at all? If the answers are, respectively, yes and no, then procreative liberty gives its blessing.

An approach centered on human flourishing requires much more. It begins with reflections on parents and children, on the values served by and intrinsic to this relationship, and on the significance of the proposed act, practice, or policy for the flourishing of children and parents. This is not a simple or easy task. It's more like a complex life-long inquiry.

The process is not mysterious, however. We must reflect on the values that are most important and most widely shared for parents, children, and families; on what makes for good lives for children, women, and men. There will not be one and only one morally defensible account of human flourishing. But not all accounts will be equally convincing. Some seek fulfillment and pleasure through tyranny and oppression or by inflicting physical or emotional cruelty, by employing manipulation and deceit, resulting in emotional emptiness. If someone wishes to defend that as a morally desirable form of human flourishing, let them try.

An insightful analysis will also acknowledge that institutions and practices shape the possibilities for flourishing—or its negation. The shaping factors include law and public policy of course, but also culture, economic circumstances, and professional norms. We must consider the implications of whatever choice confronts us for each of these factors, just as we ask how those factors themselves give shape to that choice—and how they might be refashioned to support human flourishing more vigorously.

Thinking about the Nash case by attending to values, flourishing, and context compels us to ask difficult questions. Does preimplantation testing and selection in this instance support or undermine the values central to parents and children? Will it strengthen that family's prospects for flourishing, or erode them? What effect will this case have on practices and policies in preimplantation genetic testing?

Each of these questions deserves extended reflection, more than I can provide here. My sense is that, in the end, we would conclude that the Nash family's choice was an ethically defensible action, born in compassion for the suffering of one child, and not an effort to exert excessive control over the traits of another. We could come to a very different conclusion about parents wanting to impose their preferences for less compelling ends. By contrast, procreative liberty has difficulty summoning the ethical will to curb the indulgence of almost any parental whim. That is a vitally important difference.

What are families for? This is the question we must ask when we think about the ethics of reproductive technologies. Choice and control are to be valued, but not limitlessly, and not as decisive moral panaceas. Choice is not the universal moral solvent, dissolving all moral dilemmas. We should turn first to that which shapes our lives and gives them meaning, and especially to those enduring relationships of mutual caring that grow between parents and children. Those relationships occupy crucial places in the grand tapestries of images and narratives that depict our richest and fullest images of human flourishing, as well as human failure, cruelty, and misery. When we avert our gaze from those tapestries, we blind ourselves to what ought to be our starting point for thinking insightfully about ethical issues in creating children.

NOTES

1. J.A. Robertson, *Children of Choice: Freedom and the New Reproductive Technologies* (Princeton, N.J.: Princeton University Press, 1994).

2. Kristen Luker describes these views, and the impact of recognizing that other people held quite different ones, on activists in both the pro-choice and right-to-life movements in *Abortion and the Politics of Motherhood* (Berkeley, Calif.: University of California Press, 1984).

3. J. Boswell, *The Kindness of Strangers: The Abandonment of Children in Western Europe from Late Antiquity to the Renaissance* (New York: Pantheon Press, 1988), at 37–38.

4. Quoted in S.N. Randolph, *The Domestic Life of Thomas Jefferson* (New York: Frederick Ungar, 1958).

5. T.H. Murray, *The Worth of a Child* (Berkeley, Calif.: University of California Press, 1996).

10

Mom, Dad, Clone: Implications for Reproductive Privacy

Lori B. Andrews

On 5 July 1996 a sheep named Dolly was born in Scotland, the result of the transfer of the nucleus of an adult mammary tissue cell to the enucleated egg cell of an unrelated sheep, and gestation in a third, surrogate mother sheep. (1) Although for the past ten years scientists have routinely cloned sheep and cows from embryo cells, (2) this was the first cloning experiment that apparently succeeded using the nucleus of an adult cell. (3)

Shortly after the report of the sheep cloning was published, President Clinton instituted a ban on federal funding for human cloning, (4) and asked the National Bioethics Advisory Commission (NBAC) to analyze the scientific, legal, and ethical status of human cloning and to make policy recommendations. In June 1997 NBAC recommended the passage of a federal statute that would, for a period of three to five years, ban the implantation of embryos created through human cloning, whether using private or public funding. President Clinton forwarded a bill to Congress prohibiting creating children through human cloning in the United States for at least five years.

If such a law were passed, it might be challenged as violating an individual's or a couple's right to create a biologically related child. This article explores whether such a right exists and whether, even if it does, a ban on creating children through cloning should nonetheless be upheld.

THE RIGHT TO MAKE REPRODUCTIVE DECISIONS

The right to make decisions about whether to bear children is constitutionally protected under the constitutional right to privacy (5) and the constitutional right to liberty. (6) The U.S. Supreme Court in 1992 reaffirmed the "recognized protection accorded to liberty relating to intimate relationships, the family, and decisions about whether to bear and beget a child." (7) Early decisions protected married couples' right to privacy to make procreative decisions, but later decisions focussed on individuals' rights as well. The U.S. Supreme Court, in *Eisenstadt v. Baird*, (8) stated, "if the right of privacy means anything, it is the right of the *individual*, married or single, to be free from unwarranted governmental intrusion into matters so fundamentally affecting a person as the decision whether to bear or beget a child." (9)

A federal district court has indicated that the right to make procreative decisions encompasses the right of an infertile couple to undergo medically assisted reproduction, including in vitro fertilization and the use of a donated embryo. (10) *Lifchez v. Hartigan* (11) held that a ban on research on conceptuses was unconstitutional because it impermissibly infringed upon a woman's fundamental right to privacy. Although the Illinois statute banning embryo and fetal research at issue in the case permitted in vitro fertilization, it did not allow embryo donation, embryo freezing, or experimental prenatal diagnostic procedures. The court stated:

> It takes no great leap of logic to see that within the cluster of constitutionally protected choices that includes the right to have access to contraceptives, there must be included within that cluster the right to submit to a medical procedure that may bring about, rather than prevent, pregnancy. Chorionic villi sampling is similarly protected. The cluster of constitutional choices that includes the right to abort a fetus within the first trimester must also include the right to submit to a procedure designed to give information about that fetus which can then lead to a decision to abort. (12)

Procreative freedom has been found to protect individuals' and couples' decisions to use contraception, abortion, and existing reproductive technology. Some commentators argue that the U.S. Constitution similarly protects the right to create a child through cloning.

There are a variety of scenarios in which such a right might be asserted. If both members of a couple are infertile, they may wish to clone one or the other of themselves. (13) If one member of the couple has a genetic disorder that the couple does not wish to pass on to a child, they could clone the unaffected member of the couple. In addition, if both husband and wife are carriers of a debilitating recessive genetic disease and are unwilling to run the 25% risk of bearing a child with the disorder, they may seek to clone one or the other of them. (14) This may be the only way in which the couple will be willing to have a child that will carry on their genetic line.

Even people who could reproduce coitally may desire to clone for a variety of reasons. People may want to clone themselves, deceased or living loved ones, or individuals with favored traits. A wealthy childless individual may wish to clone himself or herself to have an heir or to continue to control a family business. Parents who are unable to have another child may want to clone their dying child. (15) This is similar to the current situation in which a couple whose daughter died is making arrangements to have a cryopreserved in vitro embryo created with her egg and donor sperm implanted in a surrogate mother in an attempt to recreate their daughter. (16)

Additionally, an individual or couple might choose to clone a person with favored traits. Respected world figures and celebrities such as Mother Teresa, Michael Jordan, and Michelle Pfeiffer have been suggested as candidates for cloning. Less well-known individuals could also be cloned for specific traits. For example, people with a high pain threshold or resistance to radiation could be cloned. (17) People who can perform a particular job well, such as soldiers, might be cloned. (18) One biologist suggested cloning legless men for the low gravitational field and cramped quarters of a spaceship. (19)

Cloning also offers gay individuals a chance to procreate without using nuclear DNA from a member of the opposite sex. Clone Rights United Front, a group of gay activists, based in New York, have been demonstrating against a proposed New York law that would ban nuclear transplantation research and human cloning. They oppose such a ban because they see human cloning as a significant means of legitimizing "same-sex reproduction."(20) Randolfe Wicker founded the Clone Rights United Front in order to pressure legislators not to ban human cloning research because he sees nuclear transplantation cloning as an inalienable reproductive right." (21) Wicker stated, "We're fighting for research, and we're defending people's reproductive rights. . . . I realize my clone would be my identical twin, and my identical twin has a right to be born." (22)

Ann Northrop, a columnist for the New York gay newspaper LGNY, says that nuclear transplantation is enticing to lesbians because it offers them a means of reproduction and has the potential of giving women complete control over reproduction." (23) "This is sort of the final nail in men's coffins," she says. "Men are going to have a very hard time justifying their existence on this planet, I think. Maybe women may not let men reproduce." (24)

The strongest claim for procreative freedom is that made by infertile individuals, for whom this is the only way to have a child with a genetic link to them. However, the number of people who will actually need cloning is quite limited. Many people can be helped by in vitro fertilization and its adjuncts; others are comfortable using a donated gamete. In all the other instances of creating a child through cloning, the individual is biologically able to have a child of his or her own, but is choosing not to because he or she prefers to have a child with certain traits. This made-to-order child-making is less compelling than the infertility scenario. Moreover, there is little legal basis to suggest that a person's procreative freedom includes a right to procreate using *someone else's* DNA, such as relatives, or a celebrity. Courts are particularly unlikely to find that parents have a right to clone their young child. Procreative freedom is not a predatory right that would provide access to another individual's DNA.

The right of procreation is likely to be limited to situations in which an individual is creating a biologically related child. It could be argued that cloning oneself invokes that right to an even greater degree than normal reproduction. As lawyer Francis Pizzulli points out, "[i]n comparison with the parent who contributes half of the sexually reproduced child's genetic formula, the clonist is conferred with more than the requisite degree of biological parenthood, since he is the sole genetic parent." (25)

John Robertson argues that cloning is not qualitatively different from the practice of medically assisted reproduction and genetic selection that is currently occurring. (26) Consequently, he argues that "cloning . . . would appear to fall within the fundamental freedom of married couples, including infertile married couples to have biologically related offspring." (27) Similarly, June Coleman argues that the right to make reproductive decisions includes the right to decide in what manner to reproduce, including reproduction through, or made possible by, embryo cryopreservation and embryo twinning. (28) This argument could also be applied to nuclear transplantation by saying that a ban on cloning as a method of reproduction is tantamount to the state denying one's right to reproductive freedom.

In contrast, George Annas argues that cloning does not fall within the constitutional protection of reproductive decisions. "Cloning is replication, not reproduction, and represents a difference in kind, not in degree in the way humans continue the species." (29) He explains that "[t]his change in kind in the fundamental way in which humans can 'reproduce' represents such a challenge to human dignity and the potential devaluation of human life (even comparing the 'original' to the 'copy' in terms of which is to be more valued) that even the search for an analogy has come up empty handed." (30)

The process and resulting relationship created by cloning is profoundly different from that created through normal reproduction or even from that created through reproductive technologies such as in vitro fertilization, artificial insemination, or surrogate motherhood. In even the most high-tech reproductive technologies available, a mix of genes occurs to create an individual with a genotype that has never before existed on earth. In the case of twins, two such individuals are created. Their futures are open and the distinction between themselves and their parents is acknowledged. In the case of cloning, however, the genotype has already existed. Even though it is clear that the individual will develop into a person with different traits because of different social, environmental, and generational influences, there is evidence that the fact that he or she has a genotype that already existed will affect how the resulting clone is treated by himself, his family, and social institutions.

In that sense, cloning is sufficiently distinct from traditional reproduction or alternative reproduction to not be considered constitutionally protected. It is not a process of genetic mix, but of genetic duplication. It is not reproduction, but a sort of recycling, where a single individual's genome is made into someone else.

ASSUMING CONSTITUTIONAL PROTECTION

Let us assume, though, that courts were willing to make a large leap and find that the constitutional privacy and liberty protections of reproduction encompass cloning. If a constitutional right to clone was recognized, any legislation that would infringe unduly upon this fundamental right would be subject to a "strict standard" of judicial review. (31) Legislation prohibiting the ability to clone or prohibiting research would have to further a compelling interest in the least restrictive manner possible in order to survive this standard of review. (32)

The potential physical and psychological risks of cloning an entire individual are sufficiently compelling to justify banning the procedure. There are many physical risks to the resulting child. Of 277 attempts, only one sheep lived. The high rate of laboratory deaths may suggest that cloning in fact damages the DNA of a cell. In addition, scientists urge that Dolly should be closely monitored for abnormal genetic anomalies that did not kill her as a fetus but may have long-term harmful effects. (33)

For example, all of the initial frog cloning experiments succeeded only to the point of the amphibian's tadpole stage. (34) In addition, some of the tadpoles were grossly malformed. Initial trials in human nuclear transplantation could also meet with disastrous results. Ian Wilmut and National Institutes of Health director Harold Varmus, testifying before Congress, specifically raised the concern that cloning technology is not scientifically ready to be applied to humans, even if it were permitted, because there are technical questions that can only be answered by continued animal research. (35) Dr. Wilmut is specifically concerned with the ethical issue that would be raised by any "defective births," which may be likely to occur if nuclear transplantation is attempted with humans. (36)

In addition, if all the genes in the adult DNA are not properly reactivated, there might be a problem at a later developmental stage in the resulting clone.

(37) Some differentiated cells rearrange a subset of their genes. For example, immune cells rearrange some of their genes to make surface molecules. (38) That rearrangement could cause physical problems for the resulting clone.

Also, because scientists do not fully understand the cellular aging process, scientists do not know what 'age' or 'genetic clock' Dolly inherited. (39) On a cellular level, when the *Nature* article was published about her, was she a normal seven-month-old lamb, or was she six years old (the age of the mammary donor cell)? (40) Colin Stewart believes that Dolly's cells most likely are set to the genetic clock of the nucleus donor, and therefore are comparable to those of her six-year-old progenitor. (41) One commentator stated that if the hypotheses of a cellular, self-regulating genetic clock are correct, clones would be cellularly programmed to have much shorter life spans than the "original," which would seriously undermine many of the benefits that have been set forth in support of cloning—mostly agricultural justifications—and would psychologically lead people to view cloned animals and humans as short-lived, disposable copies. (42) This concern for premature aging has led Dr. Sherman Elias, a geneticist and obstetrician at the Baylor College of Medicine, to call for further animal testing of nuclear transplantation as a safeguard to avoid subjecting human clones to premature aging and the potential harms associated with aged cells. (43)

The hidden mutations that may be passed on by using an adult cell raise concerns as well. Mutations are "a problem with every cell, and you don't even know where to check for them," notes Ralph Brinster of the University of Pennsylvania. (44) "If a brain cell is infected with a mutant skin gene, you would not know because it would not affect the way the cell develops because it is inactive. If you choose the wrong cell, then mutations would become apparent." (45)

WHEN PHYSICAL RISKS DECLINE

The proposed federal bill would put a five-year moratorium on creating a child through cloning. During that time period, though, the physical risks of cloning will probably diminish. Animal researchers around the world are rushing to try the Wilmut technique in a range of species. If cloning appeared to be physically safe and reached a certain level of efficiency, should it then be permissible in humans?

The NBAC recommendations left open the possibility of continuing the ban on human cloning based on psychological and social risks. (46) The notion of replicating existing humans seems to fundamentally conflict with our legal system, which emphatically protects individuality and uniqueness. (47)

Banning procreation through nuclear transplantation is justifiable in light of the sanctity of the individual and personal privacy notions that are found in different constitutional amendments, and protected by the Fourteenth Amendment. (48)

The clone has lost the ability to control disclosure of intimate personal information. A ban on cloning would "preserve the uniqueness of man's personality and thus safeguard the islands of privacy which surround individuality." (49) These privacy rights are implicated through a clone's right to "retain and control the disclosure of personal information—foreknowledge of the clonant's genetic predispositions." (50) Catherine Valerio Barrad argues that courts should recognize a privacy interest in one's DNA because science is increasingly able to decipher and gather personal information from one's genetic code. (51) The fear that potential employers and health insurers may use one's private genetic information discriminatorily is not only a problem for the original DNA possessor, but any clone "made" from that individual. (52) Even in cases in which the donor waives his privacy rights and releases genetic information about himself, the privacy rights of the clone are necessarily implicated due to the fact that the clone possesses the same nucleic genetic code. (53) This runs afoul of principles behind the Fifth Amendment's protection of a "person's ability to regulate the disclosure of information about himself." (54)

If a cloned person's genetic progenitor is a famous musician or athlete, parents may exert an improper amount of coercion to get the child to develop those talents. True, the same thing may happen—to a lesser degree—now, but the cloning scenario is more problematic. A parent might force a naturally conceived child to practice piano hours on end, but will probably eventually give up if the child seems disinterested or tone deaf. More fervent attempts to develop the child's musical ability will occur if the parents chose (or even paid for) nuclear material from a talented pianist. And pity the poor child who is the clone of a famous basketball player. If he breaks his kneecap at age ten, will his parents consider him worthless? Will he consider himself a failure?

In attempting to cull out from the resulting child the favored traits of the loved one or celebrity who has been cloned, the social parents will probably limit the environmental stimuli that the child is exposed to. The pianist's clone might not be allowed to play baseball or just hang out with other children. The clone of a dead child might not be exposed to food or experiences that the first child had rejected. The resulting clone may be viewed as being in a type of "genetic bondage" (55) with improper constraints on his or her freedom.

Some scientists argue that this possibility will not come to pass because everyone knows that a clone will be different from the original. The NBAC report puts it this way: "Thus the idea that one could make through somatic cell nuclear transfer a team of Michael Jordans, a physics department of Albert Einsteins, or an opera chorus of Pavarottis, is simply false." (56) But this overlooks the fact that we are in an era of genetic determinism, in which newspapers daily report the gene for this or that and top scientists tell us that we are a packet of genes unfolding.

James Watson, co-discoverer of deoxyribonucleic acid (DNA) and the first director of the Human Genome Project, has stated, "We used to think our fate was in the stars. Now we know, in large measure, our fate is in our genes." (57) Harvard zoologist Edward O. Wilson asserts that the human brain is not *tabula rasa* later filled in by experience but, "an exposed negative waiting to be slipped into developer fluid." (58) Genetics is alleged to be so important by some scientists that it caused psychiatrist David Reiss at George Washington University to declare that "the Cold War is over in the nature and nurture debate." (59)

Whether or not this is true, parents may raise the resulting clone as if it were true. After all, the only reason people want to clone is to assure that the child has a certain genetic makeup. Thus it seems absurd to think they will forget about that genetic makeup once the child comes into being. Elsewhere in our current social policies, though, we limit parents' genetic foreknowledge of their children because we believe it will improperly influence their rearing practices.

Cloning could undermine human dignity by threatening the replicant's sense of self and sense of autonomy. A vast body of developmental psychology research has signalled the need of children to have a sense of an independent self. This might be less likely to occur if they were the clones of a member of the couple raising them or of previous children who died.

The replicant individual may be made to feel that he is less of a free agent. Laurence Tribe argues that if one's genetic makeup is subject to prior determination, "one's ability to conceive of oneself as a free and rational being entitled to resist various social claims may gradually weaken and might finally disappear altogether." (60) Under such an analysis, it does not matter whether genetics actually determines a person's characteristics. Having a predetermined genetic makeup can be limiting if the person rearing the replicant and/or the replicant believes in genetic determinism. (61) In addition, there is much research on the impact of genetic information that demonstrates that a person's genetic foreknowledge about himself or herself (whether negative or positive) can threaten that individual's self-image, harm his or her relationships with family members, and cause social institutions to discriminate against him or her. (62)

Even though parents have a constitutional right to make childrearing decisions similar to their constitutional right to make childbearing decisions, parents do not have a right to receive genetic information about their children that is not of immediate medical benefit. The main concern is that a child about whom genetic information is known in advance will be limited in his or her horizons. A few years ago, a mother entered a Huntington disease testing facility with her two young children. "I'd like you to test my children for the HD gene," she said. "Because I only have enough money to send one to Harvard." (63) That request and similar requests to test young girls for the breast cancer gene or other young children for carrier status for recessive genetic disorders raise concerns about whether parents' genetic knowledge about their child will cause them to treat that child differently. A variety of studies have suggested that there may be risks to giving parents such information.

"'Planning for the future,' perhaps the most frequently given reason for testing, may become 'restricting the future' (and also the present) by shifting family resources away from a child with a positive diagnosis," wrote Dorothy Wertz, Joanna Fanos, and Philip Reilly, in an article in the *Journal of the American Medical Association*. (64) Such a child "can grow up in a world of limited horizons and may be psychologically harmed even if treatment is subsequently found for the disorder." (65) A joint statement by the American Society of Human Genetics (ASHG) and the American College of Medical Genetics (ACMG) notes, "Presymptomatic diagnosis may preclude insurance coverage or may thwart long term goals such as advanced education or home ownership." (66)

The possibility that genetic testing of children can lead to a dangerous self-fulfilling prophecy led to the demise of one study involving testing children. Harvard researchers proposed to test children to see if they had the XYY chromosomal complement, which had been linked (by flimsy evidence) to criminality. They proposed to study the children for decades to see if those with that genetic makeup were more likely to engage in a crime than those without it. They intended to tell the mothers which children had XYY. Imagine the effect of that information—on the mother, and on the child. Each time the child took his little brother's toy, or lashed out in anger at a playmate, the mother might freeze in horror at the idea that her child's genetic predisposition was unfolding itself. She might intervene when other mothers would normally not, and thus distort the rearing of her child.

Because of the potential psychological and financial harm that genetic testing of children may cause, a growing number of commentators and advisory bodies have recommended that parents not be able to learn genetic information about their children. The Institute of Medicine Committee on Assessing Genetic Risks recommended that "in the clinical setting, children generally be tested only for disorders for which a curative or preventive treatment exists and should be instituted at that early stage. Childhood screening is not appropriate for carrier status, untreatable childhood diseases, and late-onset diseases that cannot be prevented or forestalled by early treatment." (67) The American Society of Human Genetics and American College of Medical Genetics made similar recommendations.

A cloned child will be a child who is likely to be exposed to limited experiences and limited opportunities. Even if he or she is cloned from a person who has favored traits, he may not get the benefit of that heritage. His environment might not provide him with the drive that made the original succeed. Or so many clones may be created from the favored original that their value and opportunities may be lessened. (If the entire NBA consisted of Michael Jordan clones, the game would be far less interesting and each individual less valuable.) In addition, even individuals with favored traits may have genes associated with diseases that could lead to insurance discrimination against the individuals cloned. If Jordan died young of an inheritable cardiac disorder, his clones would find their futures restricted. Banning cloning would be in keeping with philosopher Joel Feinberg's analysis that children have a right to an "open future." (68)

Some commentators argue that potential psychological and social harms from cloning are too speculative to provide the foundation for a government ban. Elsewhere, I have argued that speculative harms do not provide a sufficient reason to ban reproductive arrangements such as in vitro fertilization or surrogate motherhood. (69) But the risks of cloning go far beyond the potential psychological risks to the original whose expectations are not met in the cloning, or the risks to the child of having an unusual family arrangement if the original was not one of his or her rearing parents.

The risk here is of hubris, of abuse of power. Cloning represents the potential for "[a]buses of the power to control another person's destiny—both psychological and physical—of an unprecedented order." (70) Francis Pizzulli points out that legal discussions of whether the replicant is the property of the cloned individual, the same person as the cloned individual, or a resource for organs all show how easily the replicant's own autonomy can be swept aside. (71)

In that sense, maybe the best analogy to cloning is incest. Arguably, reproductive privacy and liberty are threatened as much by a ban on incest as by a ban on cloning. Arguably the harms are equally speculative. Yes, incest creates certain potential physical risks to the offspring, due to the potential for lethal recessive disorders to occur. But no one seriously thinks that this physical risk is the reason we ban incest. Arguably a father and daughter could avoid that risk by contracepting or agreeing to have prenatal diagnosis and abort affected fetuses. There might even be instances in which, because of their personalities, there is no psychological harm to either party.

Despite the fact that risks are speculative—and could be counterbalanced in many cases by other measures—we can ban incest because it is about improper parental power over children. We should ban the cloning of human beings through somatic cell nuclear transfer—even if physical safety is established—for that same reason.

NOTES

This article is based in part on a background paper commissioned from the author by the National Bioethics Advisory Commission.

1. Specter M, Kolata G. A new creation: the path to cloning—a special report. *New York Times* 1997; Mar 3:A1.

2. In 1993, embryologists at George Washington University split human embryos, making twins and triplets. See Sawyer K. Researchers clone human embryo cells; work is small step in aiding infertile. *Washington Post* 1993;Oct 25:A4. These embryos were not implanted into a woman for gestation. This procedure is distinguishable from cloning by nuclear transfer.

3. Begley S. Little lamb, who made thee? *Newsweek* 1997;Mar 10:53–7. See also Wilmut I, Schnieke AE, McWhir J, Kind AJ, Campbell KHS. Viable offspring derived from fetal and adult mammalian cells. *Nature* 1997;385:810–3.

4. Transcript of Clinton remarks on cloning. *U.S. Newswire* 1997;Mar 4.

5. E.g., *Griswold v. Connecticut*, 381 U.S. 379 (1965); *Eisenstadt v. Baird*, 405 U.S. 438 (1972).

6. *Planned Parenthood v. Casey*, 505 U.S. 833, 112 S.Ct. 2791 (1992).

7. *Planned Parenthood v. Casey*, 505 U.S. 833, 112 S.Ct. 2791, 2810 (1992).

8. *Eisenstadt v. Baird*, 405 U.S. 438 (1972).

9. *Eisenstadt v. Baird*, 405 U.S. 438, 453 (1972).

10. *Lifchez v. Hartigan*, 735 F.Supp. 1361 (N.D. Ill), aff'd without opinion, *sub nom.*; *Scholberg v. Lifchez*, 914 F.2d 260 (7ᵗʰ Cir. 1990), cert. denied, 111 S.Ct. 787 (1991),

11. See note 10, *Lifchez v. Harfigan* 1991.

12. See note 10, *Lifchez v. Hartigan* 1991:1377 (citations omitted). The court also held that the statute was impermissibly vague because of its failure to define "experiment" or "therapeutic" (at 1376).

13. See Wray H, Sheler JL, Watson T. The world after cloning. *U.S. News & World Report* 1997; Mar 10:59.

14. Katz J. *Experimentation with Human Beings* 977 (1972).

15. Gaylin W. We have the awful knowledge to make exact copies of human beings. *New York Times* 1997;Mar 5:48.

16. Kolata G. Medicine's troubling bonus: surplus of human embryos. *New York Times* 1997;Mar 16:1. "Fox on Trends," Fox Television Broadcast, 19 March 1997.

17. Haldane JBS. "Biological possibilities for the human species in the next thousand years", in Wolstenholme G, ed. *Man and His Future*. London: Churchill, 1963:337. Cited in Pizzulli FC. Asexual reproduction and genetic engineering: a constitutional assessment of the technology of cloning [Note]. *Southern California Law Review* 1974;47:490, n. 66.

18. Fletcher J. Ethical aspects of genetic controls. *New England Journal of Medicine* 1971;285:779.

19. See note 17, Pizzulli 1974:520.

20. Manning A. Pressing a 'right' to clone humans, some gays foresee reproduction option. *USA Today* 1997;Mar 6:Dl.

21. See note 20, Manning 1997; see also Schilinger L. Postcard from New York. *The Independent* [London] 1997;Mar 16:2.

22. See note 21, Schilinger 1997.

23. See note 20, Manning 1997.

24. See note 21, Schilinger 1997.

25. See note 17, Pizzulli 1974:550, Charles Strom, director of genetics and the DNA laboratory at Illinois Masonic Medical Center, argues that the high rate of embryo death that has occurred in animal cloning should not dissuade people from considering cloning as a legitimate reproductive technique. Strom points out that all new reproductive technologies have been marred by high failure rates, and that it is just a matter of time before cloning could be as economically efficient as any other form of artificial reproduction. See Stolberg S. Sheep clone researcher calls for caution science. *Los Angeles Times* 1997;Mar 1:AI8.

26. Robertson J. Statement to the National Bioethics Advisory Commission. 14 March 1997:83. This seems to be a reversal of Robertson's earlier position that cloning "may deviate too far from prevailing conception of what is valuable about reproduction to count as a protected reproductive experience. At some point attempts to control the entire genome of a new person pass beyond the central experiences of identity and meaning that make reproduction a valued experience." Robertson J. *Children of Choice: Freedom and the New Reproductive Technologies*. Princeton, New Jersey: Princeton University Press, 1994:169.

27. See note 26, Robertson 1994.

28. See Coleman J. Playing God or playing scientist: a constitutional analysis of laws banning embryological procedures. *Pacific Law Journal* 1996;27:1351.

29. Annas GJ. Human cloning. *ABA journal* 1997;83:80–81.

30. Annas GJ. Testimony on scientific discoveries and cloning: challenges for public policy. Subcommittee on Public Health and Safety, Committee on Labor and Human Resources, United States Senate. 12 March 1977:4.

31. See, e.g., *Griswold v. Connecticut*, 381 U.S. 479 (1965); *Eisenstadt v. Baird*, 405 U.S. 438 (1972); *Roe v. Wade*, 410 U.S. 113 (1973); *Planned Parenthood of Southern Pennsylvania v. Casey*, 505 U.S. 833 (1992).

32. See note 10, *Lifchez v. Hartigan*.

33. See Nash JM. The age of cloning. *Time* 1997;Mar 10:62–65; see also Spotts PN, Marquand R. A lamb ignites a debate on the ethnics of cloning. *Christian Science Monitor* 1997;Feb. 26:3.

34. See The law and medicine. *The Economist* 1997;Mar 1:59; see also note 17, Pizzulli 1974:484.

35. See Recer P. Sheep cloner says cloning people would be inhumane. *Associated Press* 1997;Mar 12. Reported testimony of Dr. Ian Wilmut and of Dr. Harold Varmus before the Senate on 12 March 1997 regarding the banning of human cloning research.

36. See note 35, Recer 1997. Comments of Dr. Ian Wilmut, testifying that as of yet he does not know of "any reason why we would want to copy a person. I personally have still not heard of a potential use of this technique to produce a new person that I would find ethical or acceptable."

37. Tilghman S. Statement to National Bioethics Advisory Commission, 13 March 1997:173.

38. See note 37, Tilghman 1997:147.

39. See note 35, Recer 1997.

40. See note 35, Recer 1997; see also note 33, Nash 1997:62–65.

41. See note 35, Recer 1997; Laurence J, Hornsby M. Warning on human clones. *Times* [London] 1997;Feb 23. Whatever next? *The Economist* 1997;Mar 1:79 (discussing the problems associated with having mitochondria of egg interact with donor cell).

42. Hello Dolly. *The Economist* 1997;Mar 1:17, discussing the pros and cons of aging research that could result from nuclear transplantation cloning; cf. Monmaney T. Prospect of human cloning gives birth to volatile issues. *Los Angeles Times* 1997;Mar 2:A2.

43. See note 42, Monmaney 1997.

44. See note 33, Nash 1997.

45. See note 33, Nash 1997; see also note 37, Tilghman 1997:145.

46. National Bioethics Advisory Commission. *Cloning Human Beings: Report and Recommendations of the National Bioethics Advisory Commission*. Rockville, Maryland: National Bioethics Advisory Commission, 1997:9.

47. Mauro T. Sheep clone prompts U.S. panel review. *USA Today* 1997;Feb 25:Al.

48. See note 17, Pizzulli 1974:502.

49. See note 17, Pizzulli 1974:512.

50. See note 17, Pizzulli 1974. See also Amer MS, Breaking the mold: human embryo cloning and its implications for a right to individuality. *UCLA Law Review* 1996;4:1666.

51. Valerio Barrad CM. Genetic information and property theory [Comment]. *Northwestern University Law Review* 1993;87:1050.

52. See note 51, Valerio Barrad 1993.

53. See note 51, Valerio Barrad 1993.

54. See note 50, Amer 1996.

55. See note 17, Pizzulli 1974.

56. See note 46, National Bioethics Advisory Commission 1997:33.

57. Jaroff L. The gene hunt. *Time* 1989;Mar 20:63.

58. Wolfe T. Sorry, but your soul just died. *Forbes* ASAP 1996;Dec 2:212.

59. Mann CC. Behavioral genetics in transition. *Science* 1994;264:1686.

60. Tribe L. Technology assessment and the fourth discontinuity: the limits of instrumental rationality *Southern California Law Review* 1973;46:648.

61. There is much evidence of the widespread belief in genetic determinism. See, e.g., Nelkin D, Lindee MS, *The DNA Mystique: The Gene as Cultural Icon*. New York: W.H. Freeman & Company, 1995.

62. For a review of the studies, see Andrews LB. Prenatal screening and the culture of motherhood. *Hastings Law Journal* 1996;47:967.

63. Wexler N. Clairvoyance and caution: repercussions from the Human Genome Project. In Kevles DJ, Hood L. *The Code of Codes: Scientific and Social Issues in the Human Genome Project*. Cambridge, Massachusetts: Harvard University Press, 1992:211–43, 233.

64. Wertz D, Fanos J, Reilly P. Genetic testing for children and adolescents: who decides? *JAMA* 1994;274:878.

65. See note 64, Wertz et al. 1994. Similarly, the ASHG/ACMG Statement notes: "Expectations of others for education, social relationships and/or employment may be significantly altered when a child is found to carry a gene associated with a late-onset disease or susceptibility. Such individuals may not be encouraged to reach their full potential, or they may have difficulty obtaining education or employment if their risk for early death or disability is revealed." American Society of Human Genetics and American College of Medical Genetics. Points to consider: ethical, legal, and psychosocial implications of genetic testing in children and adolescents. *American Journal of Human Genetics* 1995;57:1233–41, 1236.

66. See note 65, ASHG/ACMG 1995.

67. Andrews LB, Fullarton JE, Holtzman NA, Motulsky AG, eds. *Assessing Genetic Risks: Implications for Health and Social Policy*. Washington, D.C.: National Academy of Sciences, 1994:276.

68. See note 46, National Bioethics Advisory Commission 1997:67.

69. Andrews LB. Surrogate motherhood: the challenge for feminists. *Law, Medicine & Health Care* 1988;72:16.

70. See note 17, Pizzulli 1974:497.

71. See note 17, Pizzulli 1974:492.

11

Cloned Child

J. M. Phillips

However she comes to us,
glass-engendered,
slipping from her temporary womb
like a tenement dweller
into arms kindly or clinical,
she will be ours,
bone of our bone,
blood of our blood,
and *our* predicament.
She will remind us that
all we sum up, predict, and blueprint
must still fill inexplicably with soul.
She is the subject of her voyage,
come to us from depths
we cannot hope to fathom
up the anchor-line of wonder.
Like the coming of every child
she comes announcing what otherwise
we would not know.

Index

Page numbers in italic refer to tables or figures

About the Editor

Thomas A. Shannon is professor of religion and social ethics at Worcester Polytechnic Institute. He is the author of many articles and books in Catholic social thought, bioethics, and genetics. He is coauthor with Thomas Massaro of *Catholic Perspectives on Peace and War*, with James J. Walter of *The New Genetic Medicine*, and is the editor of a series of readers in bioethics for Sheed & Ward.